Kundalini Yoga for Self-Care and Caregivers

Includes Chair Yoga Options

**IVONNE WOPEREIS &
MONIQUE SIAHAYA**

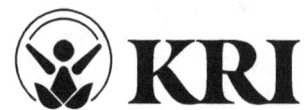

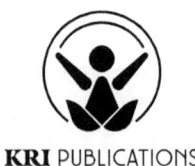

© 2023 KUNDALINI RESEARCH INSTITUTE
BY MONIQUE SIAHAYA AND IVONNE WOPEREIS
PUBLISHED BY THE KUNDALINI RESEARCH INSTITUTE
TRAINING • PUBLISHING • RESEARCH • RESOURCES
PO BOX 1819 SANTA CRUZ, NM 87532
WWW.KUNDALINIRESEARCHINSTITUTE.ORG
ISBN: 978-0-9639991-5-3
MANAGING EDITOR: MARIANA LAGE (HARISHABAD KAUR)
CONSULTING EDITOR: AMRIT SINGH KHALSA
LINE EDITOR: ONG KAR KAUR KHALSA
REVIEWER: SIRI NEEL KAUR KHALSA AND DIANA NANU
PROOFREADER: CARLOS ANDREI SIQUARA
COVER AND CREATIVE CONCEPT: FERNANDA MONTE-MOR
LAYOUT: CAROLINE GISCHEWSKI
PHOTOGRAPHY: THAMAR WEERTS AND PIM SIAHAYA
EDITORIAL ASSISTANTS: ANTONIO LARA SILVA

© Kundalini Research Institute. All teachings, yoga sets, techniques, kriyas and meditations courtesy of The Teachings of Yogi Bhajan. Reprinted with permission. Unauthorized duplication is a violation of applicable laws. ALL RIGHTS RESERVED. No part of these Teachings may be reproduced or transmitted in any form by any means, electronic or mechanical, including photocopying and recording, or by any information storage and retrieval system, except as may be expressly permitted in writing by The Teachings of Yogi Bhajan. To request permission, please write to KRI at PO Box 1819, Santa Cruz, NM 87567 or see www.kundaliniresearchinstitute.org.

The diet, exercise and lifestyle suggestions in this book come from ancient yogic traditions. Nothing in this book should be construed as medical advice. Neither the author nor the publisher shall be liable or responsible for any loss, injury, damage, allegedly arising from any information or suggestion in this book. The benefits attributed to the practice of Kundalini Yoga and meditation stem from centuries-old yogic tradition. Results will vary with individuals. Always check with your personal physician or licensed care practitioner before making any significant modification in your diet or lifestyle, to ensure that the lifestyle changes are appropriate for your personal health condition and consistent with any medication you may be taking.

This publication has received the KRI Seal of Approval. This Seal is given only to products that have been reviewed for accuracy and integrity of the sections containing the 3HO lifestyle and Kundalini Yoga as taught by Yogi Bhajan®. For more information about Kundalini Yoga as taught by Yogi Bhajan® please see www.kundaliniresearchinstitute.org.

Kundalini Yoga for Self-Care and Caregivers

Includes Chair Yoga Options

**IVONNE WOPEREIS &
MONIQUE SIAHAYA**

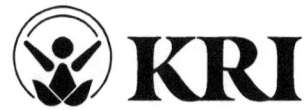

SUMMARY

INTRODUCTION	**9**
Chakras: What They Are Chakras and How To Work With Them	11
Key Points to Be Aware of Before and During Your Practice	12
Building Up Practice	13
The Posture	14
How to Start	15
The Breath	16
How to Breathe	16
Specific Breaths	16
The Kriya	17
The Body Locks	18
The Hand Positions (Mudras)	18
The Relaxation Exercise	19
How to End the Yoga Session	20
CHAPTER 1	
DEEP LISTENING	**23**
1.1 Listening Meditation	25
1.2 Kriya to Relax and Release Fear	26
1.3 Pran Bandha Mantra	38
CHAPTER 2	
HARD DECISIONS	**43**
2.1 Kriya for the Back	46
2.2 Sending Healing Thoughts Meditation	54
2.3 Meditation for Change	58
CHAPTER 3	
LOSS AND GRIEF	**61**
3.1 Meditation to Prevent Freaking Out	64
3.2 Evening Kriya	66
3.3 Kriya Removing Fear of the Future	76

CHAPTER 4
FOUNDATIONS   79
    4.1 Long and Deep Breathing   82
    4.2 Basic Spinal Energy Series   86
    4.3 Kirtan Kriya Meditation   98

CHAPTER 5
ENJOYMENT   103
    5.1 Sitali Kriya: Cooling and Calming Breath   106
    5.2 Kriya for Adrenals & Kidneys   108
    5.3 Antar Naad Mudra - Kabadshe Meditation   122

CHAPTER 6
SELF-ESTEEM   125
    6.1 Self-Care Breath: Healing Pranayam   128
    6.2 Kriya to Take Away Fear & Sadness   130
    6.3 Meditation for the Third Chakra   138

CHAPTER 7
AWARENESS   141
    7.1 Kriya for Expanding Lung Capacity   144
    7.2 Kriya to Open the Heart Center   148
    7.3 Meditation for a Calm Heart   156

CHAPTER 8
SELF EXPRESSION   161
    8.1 Kriya to Develop Command Reflex and Alertness   164
    8.2 Kriya for Intuition and Communication   174
    8.3 Meditation: Aad Naad Kriya   178
    Additional Exercise:
    Universal rules of communication   180

CHAPTER 9
PURPOSE   183

    9.1   Becoming Aware of Your Breath   186
    9.2   Kriya to Become Intuitive   188
    9.3   Meditation for Powerful Energy   194

CHAPTER 10
BELONGING   197

    10.1   Whistling Breath   200
    10.2   Kriya Foundation for Infinity   202
    10.3   Meditation into Being: I Am I Am   214

CHAPTER 11
ADDITIONAL RESOURCES
SELF-CARE KIT   219

    11.1   Warm-Up with Butterfly   222
    11.2   Movement Relaxation Series   226
    11.3   Kriya for the Electromagnetic Field   230
    11.4   Meditation for the Arcline and to Clear the Karmas   236
    11.5   Become Calm – Earth to Self   240

ABOUT THE AUTHORS   243

INTRODUCTION
—

Whatever your age or physical ability, yoga can always be used as a way to support yourself. Whenever you're stuck in a pattern in your life, yoga can help you become aware of it and figure out what you want to do about it. Breathing exercises can help you feel calmer and more connected to yourself. Mantras can focus your thoughts while also calming your mind. Yoga practice can improve your breathing ability. When you practice a series of yoga exercises with a specific effect (a kriya), it can give you more flexibility, insight into your body's systems, and awareness of your emotions. Through meditation, you learn that your thoughts do not determine your life and that you can direct your stream of thoughts and even let them pass.

The program Kundalini Yoga for Self-Care is designed for anyone who wants to support themselves through yoga and meditation. It promotes self-awareness and nurtures your understanding around your main life themes. It aids you in discovering what you truly need to support yourself. This program will help you learn more about your boundaries and about being yourself. As a result, you'll realize that you have a choice in how you respond to life's challenges. You will gain more acceptance for yourself and your situation, and the world around you will come into clearer focus. The program helps you improve physical and mental flexibility, allowing you to feel more relaxed and at ease with yourself.

The program consists of eleven chapters and addresses important life themes. Each chapter will cover a different theme. The breathing exercises, yoga sets, meditations, and, among other yoga techniques, coordinate with the life themes, promote self-care, and raise awareness about how to provide relief to life's problems. The program overview at the start of each chapter indicates which themes will be covered. The yogic techniques were chosen with care to correspond with the life themes.

Kundalini Yoga for Self-Care and Caregivers uses kundalini yoga techniques as taught by Yogi Bhajan®. You will find these techniques on the left pages (even numbers). These same techniques have been adapted to be practiced on a chair. Therefore you will find a chair version of the same yoga set or meditation on the right pages (odd numbers). Through the program, you will discover which obstacles you face in daily life. You'll learn what you can do to live with the obstacle or, if you prefer, change it. You can also share experiences with others and learn from one another, so that you realize that you are not alone.

Take a moment for yourself each day to practice one or more elements of the program in this book. You can begin by practicing 11 minutes per day. This daily practice encourages the emergence of new patterns of self-care, which in turn will benefit others as well. Once you have completed the exercises in this book, you can continue to practice some of them (or any of them) to further support yourself in the self-care journey.

This program was created for people of all ages and abilities, and it can be practiced by younger as well as older people. The pages on the left (even numbers) include yoga for practice on the mat. The pages on the right side of the book (odd numbers) include a chair yoga adaptation, which is ideal for anyone with limited mobility or in a setting where chairs are the primary mode of exercise available. Throughout the kriyas in the footnote sections, you will find extra information and adaptations for each of the exercises. Different times are indicated for each version — on the mat or on the chair. The full times apply to those who are young, healthy and in good shape. Reduced times are indicated in the correct proportions for chair yoga, which is aimed at people who are older or have health and movement limitations.

We, the authors, have both been yoga teachers and caregivers in our lives for many years. We know from personal experience how incredibly nurturing yoga can be during the often difficult process of caregiving. We have provided support to people who are looking after families and communities through our yoga groups. We have found that this additional assistance was extremely beneficial to these caregivers. When developing this program and creating the chair yoga adaptations, we researched and sought out information from various groups of people who provide care for others.

Be creative and use your intuition, when practicing yoga. Adjust times for yoga exercises to suit decreased stamina and flexibility, and encourage seniors to try only postures that they can comfortably manage.

- » Begin where you are. From a place of acceptance, an opening is created for change to take place.
- » Something is better than nothing. Each person is unique, as is their healing journey. Exercising or meditating for what appears to be a short period of time shouldn't be dismissed or undervalued.
- » A small amount goes a long way. Those experiencing health challenges should progress slowly into mastery of a few exercises rather than moving too quickly towards multiple challenges.

> Begin with warming up the body. It is important to do warm-up exercises before a kriya for people who have health issues or are getting older. These warm-ups are needed to provide grounding and also to increase circulation to the feet and lower legs.

The chapters progress by incorporating life themes that are beneficial for people who are caregivers, so that they can be supported on all levels, from energetic to physical and emotional. These life themes often have a connection with the energy centers in your body, also known as chakras. The first three chapters are concerned with life themes specific to times of difficulty and change. How, for example, do we make radical decisions? What would you do if you feel incapable of caring for your child? Or imagine that a loved one has passed away, how do we deal with grief and loss. These are all difficult moments in our life to navigate. In the subsequent seven chapters, you'll go through the seven chakras that are connected with the physical and subtle or sensitive life themes. After that, there is the final chapter with additional resources for your self-care.

Chakras: What They Are and How To Work With Them

The body is physical — we can see that. There is also a field of energy and activity that we cannot see with our own eyes. Within this field of energy there are seven important energy centers, known as the chakras. The chakras are centers of transformation and connection that influence one another through our thoughts, moods, state of health, and other bodily functions. The chakras exchange energy back and forth from gross to subtle. These chakras function like doorways to acknowledgment.

The chakras run the length of the spine, from the tailbone to the crown of our head. They are described as vortices that spin from the front to the back of the body. The bottom and top chakras spin in opposite directions, toward earth and heaven, respectively. Some people can feel chakras with their hands; they have the energy sensation of a whirlpool without water. Others may perceive them as rainbow colors. The lower five chakras are connected to the elements:

earth, water, fire, air and ether. All of the chakras are linked to archetypal life themes. As a result, each chakra is associated with a talent or a gift. The first chakra is associated with the phrase "I accept who I am"; the second with "I feel and create"; the third with "I connect myself to action"; the fourth with "I love and empathize"; the fifth with "I communicate the truth"; the sixth with "I see through my intuition"; the seventh with "I am free and I understand."

In the course of your development on this earth, your chakras can open up like a flower bud. This chakra opening doesn't always occur in the desirable order. For example, if you were not well-cared for as a baby, you may develop a dysfunction or a shadow element of your first chakra. When the energy centers are out of balance, it can cause disruptions and bring shadow elements in your life. The chakra system can bring to light the non-visible (subtle) and/or visible (physical) energy, as well as the accompanying emotions, thoughts and moods, and it can aid in the resolution of disturbances and shadow elements within a person.

Key Points to Be Aware of Before and During Your Practice

In this section, you find basic information concerning the practice of yoga, such as instructions for breath, posture and relaxation. It is recommended to carefully read the information below.

For the yoga practice, you may need:
» A natural-material mat to enhance the circulation of the electromagnetic field and keep a warm layer away from the cold floor. You can also use a stable chair.
» Clothes that are comfortable to exercise in.
» A blanket, shawl, sweater and warm socks to use during relaxation exercises.
» Make sure the space is clean and quiet, as well as well-ventilated, so that you can practice without being disturbed. A permanent spot within the house is beneficial.
» A set time to practice during the day can be helpful in building up a discipline.
» Quiet mantra music to play during relaxation exercises.

- » Allow at least two hours between meals and practicing yoga.
- » Focus on the breath during yoga practice.
- » Unless otherwise specified, it is recommended to close the eyes and focus on the Third Eye Point (in between the brows with the eyes slightly raised upward) to support the inner experience and concentration during the exercise or meditation.
- » Drink plenty of water both before and after the yoga practice. It facilitates the removal of toxins from the body more easily both during and after exercise.

A good structure for a complete yoga session includes:
- » Exercises for loosening and warming up
- » Chanting the tuning in mantra **ONG NAMO GUROO DAYV NAMO**
- » A breathing exercise
- » A kriya (set of Kundalini Yoga exercises)
- » Relaxation
- » A meditation
- » To conclude: *Long Time Sun* and *Sat Naam*

At home, you can do only a portion of a full session, such as singing the opening mantra and performing a single breathing exercise, a kriya (series of exercises), and a long deep relaxation. Even if you only practice for a few minutes, you will generate energy and set it in motion. We recommend that you always take a few moments to relax after each exercise. Always read the whole kriya or meditation before getting started.

Building Up Practice

While practicing yoga, respect your own body and use both your head and your intuition to determine the length, intensity and pace of the exercise. Experiment and find out what feels good, and don't force yourself. Pain is a signal that should not be ignored, and if you experience dizziness, you should slow down or stop. You can gradually increase your practice time, but never go beyond the maximum times specified. When you are young and in good shape, you can try the maximum times indicated, but you can also gradually increase the time of each exercise. If you're older, feeling out of shape, have disabilities, or your vitality is diminishing, don't go out of your comfort zone while practicing yoga. Build up slowly, and start with the time indicated in the chair yoga sections.

If you are unable to do the exercise as described, you can visualize it instead. Exercise at your own pace and take breaks in between. Notice how each exercise affects you; observe without judgment, relax, and keep breathing! When you allow the impact of each exercise to fall into place, you will notice an increase in body awareness.

Exercises that need to be done on both sides are typically repeated for an equal amount of time on each side, unless the instructions specify only one side or for a shorter time. Some exercises are done only on one side to achieve a specific effect.

It can be beneficial to practice an exercise, yoga series or meditation for 40 consecutive days. A 40 day time period is known in yogic tradition to be a cycle of time that affects a change in both mind and body. This daily repetition helps a new pattern or a new habit to develop. If you practice a meditation for 40 days, your subconscious will begin to release the thoughts and emotional patterns that have been holding you back. Try committing to a 40 day practice – without skipping a single day –, and observe what changes occur in how you think and feel.

The Posture

Paying attention to posture is essential in yoga. Begin by finding your comfortable seat. During each exercise, sit actively and with conscious focus. In the chair yoga version, move slightly forward to the front of the seat, without touching the back of the seat. Sit up straight and tall. Feel your feet, legs, pelvis, and sit bones. Sit between both sit bones, and don't tilt the pelvis too far back or forth. Pull a Root Lock: this is a muscular contraction in the pelvic area combined with a navel contraction. Feel your weight and the sensation of being rooted through the earth. Stretch the tailbone slightly forward. Stretch the spine up, open the chest wide, relax the shoulders, and draw the shoulder blades down, keep the neck long, and lift the back of the head slightly.

When bending forward, always bend from the hips. Pull up on the pelvic floor muscles before you begin to bend. Make sure your pelvic bone is slightly in front of your sit bones. You will feel a light pressure in the thighs.

Before turning left or right with your upper body, it is important to begin by lengthening your spine and standing tall with your upper body. It is especially important in the case of conditions of the spine to not force anything and to feel what you are actually able to do, specifically when turning and bending backward.

When bending backward, balance the tailbone by pulling it under you. Pull up on the pelvic floor muscles, elongate the spine, stretch the middle and upper part of the back, and bring your sternum up and forward. When you've finished the exercise, slowly push yourself forward and out of the backward bend.

How to Start

Before practicing a Kundalini Yoga kriya, meditation or breath, begin by chanting a mantra, which is a sound or words that give direction to your mind through repetition and rhythm. This assists you in connecting with the source of yoga, by contacting your inner wisdom, which guides and protects you.

Put your palms together, thumbs pointing upward and resting against your chest. This hand position puts you in a state of neutrality. Allow yourself to be open to the experience, take a deep breath and begin chanting the mantra **ONG NAMO GUROO DAYV NAMO**. Repeat it 2 more times. After chanting the mantra, place your hands in your lap and just inhale and exhale a few times.

The "O" sound in Ong is long, as in "go," and of short duration. The "ng" sound is long and produces a definite vibration on the roof of the mouth and the cranium. The "O" is held longer. The first syllable of Guru is pronounced as in the word "good." The second syllable rhymes with "true." The first syllable is short and the second one is long. The word Dev rhymes with "gave."

"Ong" is the infinite creative energy experienced in manifestation and activity. It is a variant of the cosmic syllable "Om," which refers to God in Its absolute or unmanifest state. "Namo" has the same root as the Sanskrit word "Namaste," which means reverent greetings. It implies bowing and reverence. Together, "Ong Namo" means "I call on the infinite creative consciousness," and it opens you to the universal consciousness that guides all action.

"Guru" is the embodiment of the wisdom that one is seeking. "Dev" means higher, subtle, or divine. It refers to the spiritual realms. "Namo," at the end of the mantra, reaffirms the humble reverence of the student. Taken together, "Guru Dev Namo" means, "I call on the divine wisdom," whereby you bow before your higher self to guide you in using the knowledge and energy given by the cosmic self.

The Breath
Breath is life. Breathing relaxes, cleanses, and brings you back to yourself, to your center. If you feel dizzy while doing a breathing exercise, stop doing this specific breath. Breathe naturally and rest for a bit. When you practice yoga and breathing exercises regularly and for a longer period of time, the dizziness should normally go away.

During the exercises, always try to inhale and exhale through the nose, unless otherwise specified. It is better for the lungs to breathe through the nose, where the air is preheated, filtered, and moistened. Sit up straight to allow your belly and chest to expand. Wear loose and comfortable clothing, especially around the waist.

How to Breathe
Sit up straight on the mat. If practicing on the chair, sit with your feet flat on the ground. Stretch the spine from your tailbone to the thoracic vertebrae, where the ribs begin, then stretch from the bottom thoracic vertebrae upward to your seventh cervical vertebra. This seventh or bottom cervical vertebra is a protrusion that you can feel when bending your head forward. Then lengthen the spine from the seventh cervical vertebra to the crown, the highest point of the skull. Feel the stretch along the length of the spine. This posture allows you to breathe more freely.

Let go of any unnecessary tension. Notice the areas of your stomach, back, shoulder, face, throat, tongue and lips. Allow the energy to flow through your body. Don't try to force anything. Allow yourself to grow at your own pace and with your own intensity. Do the breathing exercises for the allotted time; they are never done for more time than specified in the exercise.

Specific Breaths
BREATH OF FIRE. It is quick, rhythmic and continuous. Breath of Fire is powered from the Navel Point and the solar plexus. The in and out breath are equally long, without pause, with a closed mouth, and breathing through the nose. When you start, breathe in a little bit, so that the diaphragm becomes more flexible. While breathing out, the breath is powerfully pushed out through the nose, while the Navel Point and the solar plexus move inward. While breathing in, the Navel Point and solar plexus move forward again. The chest and the rest of the body remain relaxed. Do not exaggerate the belly movement while breathing. Be careful to breathe an equal amount in and out, so that the proportions are correct.

To learn Breath of Fire, place the hands on the area under the diaphragm, so that you feel the movement in this area, and you can check if the navel and solar plexus move forward while breathing in and move inward while breathing out.

Beginners may experience dizziness because it is a new and powerful breath practice or if the Breath of Fire is practiced too fast. If so, stop practicing Breath of Fire, and carry on breathing normally. You may also try practicing Breath of Fire at a slower pace at first to learn to regulate your breathing. In general the pace of the Breath of Fire is reduced for chair yoga.

CANNON BREATH. Powerful Breath of Fire through a round mouth, from the area of the solar plexus.

The Kriya

The word kriya means: action leading to a complete change. A kriya can consist of one exercise or a series of exercises. The key point is that they work on specific themes on multiple levels, including physical, mental, emotional, energetic, and spiritual. To reach the desired effect, it is necessary to practice the kriya as it is described. Do not change the sequence and the instructions for practice. Don't omit any exercise from the series or add anything. If possible, practice the original kriya with the times given for practice. If it better suits your individual needs, adapt the time intervals proportionally or practice a chair yoga adaptation.

The authors have adapted the kriyas for chair yoga, so that they can be done by elderly people with limited mobility or those with medical conditions. The goal of adapting the kriyas for chair yoga was to match the essence of the exercise or posture and the abilities of the elderly or those with limited mobility. The time intervals in the kriyas for chair yoga have been reduced proportionally to each other, for example half or a third of the original times for each exercise. The one exception is never to practice an exercise for less than one minute.

The kriyas in this book have been carefully chosen and tested. Their efficacy has been thoroughly researched and practiced as well. They have been tailored to the themes suitable for people who are providing care experience on a daily basis. If you have a medical condition that prevents you from performing an exercise, you can visualize the posture instead.

The Body Locks

Bandhas or body locks are combinations of muscle contractions and are frequently used in Kundalini Yoga. Each lock has the function of changing blood circulation, nerve pressure, and the flow of cerebrospinal fluid. They also direct the praana, the flow of psychic energy, into the main energy channels that relate to raising the Kundalini energy. They concentrate the body's energy for use in consciousness and self-healing. There are three important locks: Root Lock (*mulbandh*), Neck Lock (*jalandhar bandh*), and Diaphragm Lock (*uddiyana bandh*). When all three locks are applied simultaneously, it is called the Great Lock (*maahaabandh*).

ROOT LOCK: This is a contraction of the muscles in the pelvic floor, combined with the navel. Start by simultaneously pulling the anal sphincter in and up; then pull the area of the sex organs in the direction of the pubic bone. This feels as if you are trying to hold your water. Then pull your navel toward the spine. This pulling action is regularly applied at the end of an exercise, while holding the breath in or out to let the effect of the exercise fall into place.

NECK LOCK: Sit comfortably with your spine stretched, lift the sternum, and simultaneously stretch the back of your neck by slightly pulling your chin toward your chest. The head remains stable. The muscles of the neck and throat stay relaxed, as well as the facial muscles and the brow. Make sure not to force the head down or backward.

DIAPHRAGM LOCK: Never practice on an empty stomach and only on a full exhalation. Sit comfortably. Inhale deeply, exhale completely. Pull the navel, especially the area above the Navel Point, up toward the spine. The Navel Point is not contracted, only pulled upward. Lift the sternum. Gently push your thoracic and lumbar vertebra forward. Keep the stretch for 10 to 60 seconds but not with tension. Then let go of the contraction, gradually inhale while maintaining the Neck Lock.

GREAT LOCK: Pull all body locks at once — the Neck Lock, the Diaphragm Lock, and the Root Lock.

The Hand Positions (Mudras)

BEAR GRIP: Place the left palm facing out from the chest with the thumb down. Place the palm of the right hand facing the chest. Bring the fingers together. Curl the fingers of both hands, so the hands form a fist. This mudra is used to stimulate the heart and to intensify concentration.

BUDDHA MUDRA: Rest the left palm face-up in the lap with the right hand palm-up on top of it. Put the thumb tips together or not, based on the instructions of a particular kriya.

BUDDHI MUDRA: Place the tip of the little finger on the tip of the thumb. Practicing this opens the capacity to communicate clearly and intuitively. It also stimulates psychic development. The little finger is symbolized by Mercury for quickness and the mental power of communication.

GYAN MUDRA: The tips of the thumbs and index fingers touch, the other fingers are extended.

LOTUS MUDRA: Hold the hands in front of the Heart Center, and join the base of the hands, and the tips of the thumbs and Mercury (little) fingers with space between the palms and the other fingers spread apart.

PRANAM MUDRA: Also known as Prayer Pose. The palms of the hands are flat together to balance the positive (right or masculine) and negative (left or feminine) sides of the body.

VENUS LOCK: For working feminine, reflective energy, interlace the hands with the tip of the right thumb on the tissue between thumb and index finger. Then push the tip of the left thumb against the ball of the right thumb. For working with masculine, projective energy, the position of the thumbs and fingers is opposite, with the left little finger at the bottom and the right thumb on top.

YOGA MUDRA: Interlace the fingers behind your back with palms facing up. The elbows are bent. Tighten your pelvic floor muscles, bend forward, and bring the Heart Center towards the ground. Then stretch your arms and lift them away from your back. You can hold a scarf behind your back if necessary.

The Relaxation

Always make sure to relax after a series of exercises or a meditation. This will complete the effect of the yoga; what happens during the exercise will fall into place, and the complementary exercise and relaxation will provide balance.

Example of a guided relaxation: "Relax your feet and your hips, relax your ankles, then the calves and shins. Feel your knees and thighs as heavy and relaxed. Relax your hips and buttocks, your tailbone, your sacrum. Feel your lower back and relax into the ground. Imagine your back is very wide and long. Relax the shoulders and shoulder blades. Direct your attention to your belly, feel the warmth, and relax all the muscles of your belly. Relax your stomach and feel deeper into your abdomen. Feel your chest wide and relaxed, and feel your shoulders. Direct your attention to your hands, your fingers, relax your forearms, your elbows and your upper arms. Go from your shoulders to your neck and relax there. Feel your throat and your jaws. Feel the tongue resting in the mouth, relaxing the cheeks and your nose, the eyes and the ears. Let the forehead relax, becoming smooth and supple. Relax your hair and even the hair follicles. Try to relax your thoughts, let them go." Stay seated or lying down for up to 11 minutes — or more when indicated. You can listen to quiet mantra music.

After 11 minutes, inhale and exhale deeply a couple of times. Then move your toes and feet, followed by your fingers and hands. Move your head slowly back and forth, and stretch yourself out entirely. Still lying on the mat, do a cat stretch by stretching the arms to the sides, lift a knee into the chest and draw it across the body to lower it to the floor over the extended leg, while you turn your head in the opposite direction. Do cat stretch on the other side. Then pull the knees into the chest and roll from side to side. Rub the palms of the hands and the soles of the feet vigorously together. Then, roll over the length of the back and come back to sitting position.

How to End the Yoga Session

To end, sit up straight. Put the palms together, the thumbs are pointing up and resting against the sternum. Inhale deeply and chant the mantra **SAT NAAM** three times ("Sat" lasts 7 seconds, "Naam" 1 second). The mantra means "Truth is my name," or "my true identity." This mantra connects you with your soul and your destination.

In Kundalini yoga classes or when practicing alone, we sing a short song before chanting three long Sat Naam. The song is an inspiring prayer for the rest of your day. It says: "May the Long Time Sun Shine Upon You, All Love Surround You, And the Pure Light Within You Guide Your Way On."[1]

We hope you have a caring and nurturing journey within yourself in the pages to come. We prepared this yoga manual to inspire and support you in your self-development, self-improvement and self-care. We wish for each person who practices Kundalini Yoga for Self-care a lighter life journey ahead.

Sat Naam,
Ivonne Wopereis and Monique Siahaya
July 2022

---

[1] You can find a beautiful version of this chant on the internet or go to the Gurbani Media Center from Sikhnet at sikhnet.com/gurbani/

CHAPTER 1
Deep Listening
—

Consciously ask your intuition to show you the path.
Consciously ask your courage to face the calamity.
Ask your grace to face the insecurity.
Ask your breath of life to face depression.
Rise, rise and excel.

— YOGI BHAJAN, JUNE 30, 1994

Caregivers and those who are drawn to a focus on self-care, in particular, require an understanding of the life theme of what to do once we find ourselves in crisis. This chapter provides key resources to draw on when life begins to turn upside down. The first resource is the breath, which is the foundation of your life force, praana, which will allow you to regain control of yourself. The second is deep listening, which reveals how your rhythms and patterns change as a result of the crisis. Next we find that relaxation and letting go of fear aid in achieving stability. In order to deal with the crisis, regaining our stability is an essential resource. Finally, connecting with the higher self gives the assurance of being guided by what has always been and continues to be.

The kriyas and meditations presented in this chapter assist you in the process of becoming more aware of the life theme of handling crisis, and understanding the resources that will help you through this time. These resources are your deep listening, awareness, knowing your rhythm and patterns, connection, relaxation, and letting go of fear. These are all aspects that help you find your rootedness in your stability, while gaining flexibility to respond to change.

You begin with a listening meditation to be able to hear your needs. The breath practice in the *Listening Meditation* helps you in becoming calmer and better in connecting with yourself. The *Kriya to Relax and Release Fear* assists you physically and energetically by relaxing and letting go of fear that has been held in the body. The meditation *Pran Bandha Mantra* connects you with your higher self, enabling you to adopt a different approach to life, which is needed to progress through times of change and crisis. Sit in Easy Pose with a straight spine and a light Neck Lock.

1.1 Listening Meditation

From Dr Shanti Shanti Kaur Khalsa personal notes.

Mudra: Rest your hands on your knees or in your lap palms facing up.

Eye Focus: Closed.

Breath: Natural, deep and even. Listen calmly and deeply. Although more than one sound may occur at the same time, allow yourself to hear each sound one at a time. Let your attention move from sound to sound as you remain still, listening and identifying each one.

Time: 11 minutes.

To End: Inhale deeply, suspend your breath briefly, and exhale completely. Relax your posture and open your eyes.

ON THE CHAIR

Sit comfortably in a chair with the weight of both feet resting evenly on the ground, with a straight spine and a light Neck Lock.

Practice as described on the side.

Time: Continue for **3 minutes.**

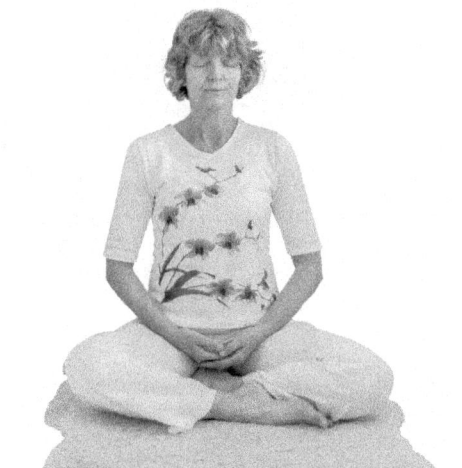
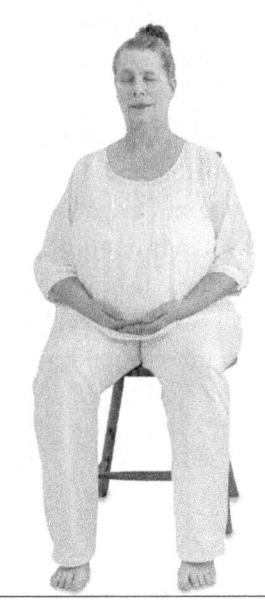

KUNDALINI YOGA FOR SELF-CARE AND CAREGIVERS

1.2 Kriya to Relax and Release Fear
Originally taught in the summer of 1983

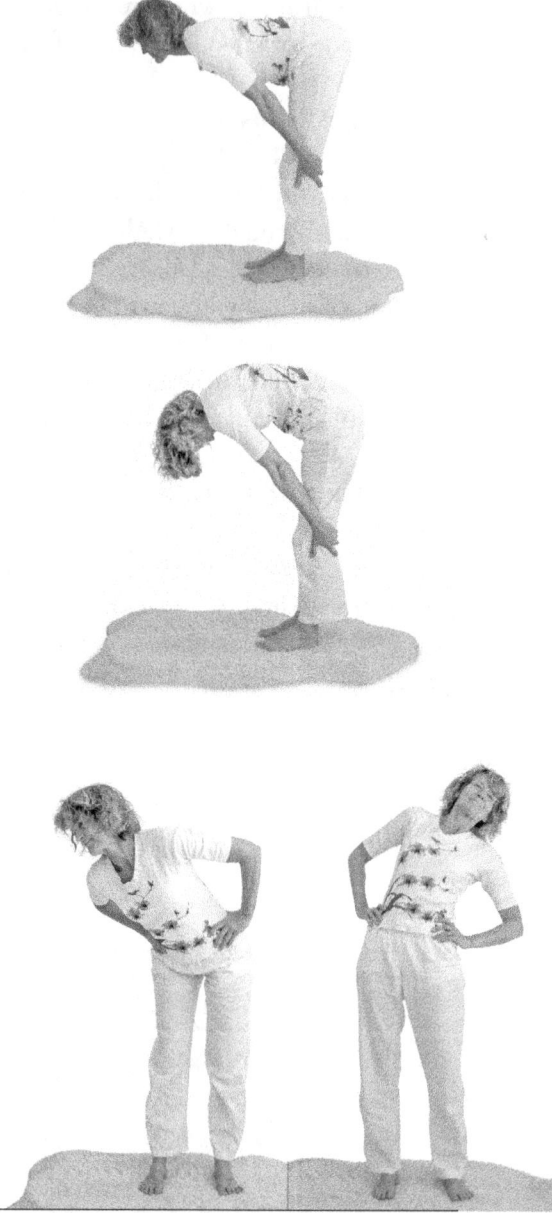

1) STANDING CAT-COW.
Stand up and bend forward from the hips, keeping the back parallel to the ground. Reach behind your legs and hold on to your calves or whatever you may reach to maintain your balance. Begin to flex the spine as in Cat-Cow Posture. Inhale and arch your back downward, lowering the belly, lifting the sternum and chin and broadening the collarbones. Keep the back of the neck long. Exhale and round your spine upward, bringing the chin to the chest. Use the hands and feet as a firm base of support for the spine. Keep the arms and legs straight. Maintain a steady rhythm for **7 minutes.**
This exercise works on the kidneys and liver.

2) STANDING TORSO CIRCLES.
Remain standing with a straight spine and a light Neck Lock. Place the hands on the hips. Rapidly rotate the torso in large circles from the hips. Continue for **9 minutes.**
This exercise rejuvenates the spleen and releases toxins from the liver.

→ continue on next page

ON THE CHAIR

1) STANDING CAT-COW.
Sit comfortably in a chair with the weight of both feet resting evenly on the ground, with a straight spine and a light Neck Lock. Bend forward from the hips while keeping the spine straight. Place the right foot on the ground and stretch the left leg straight forward. Grasp the left calf or place your hands behind the knee. Begin to flex the spine as in Cat-Cow Posture. Inhale and arch your back downward, lowering the belly, lifting the sternum and chin and broadening the collarbones. Keep the back of the neck long. Exhale and round your spine upward, bringing the chin to the chest. Keep the extended leg straight. Maintain a steady rhythm for **1 minute**, then change legs. Continue for another **1 minute**.
This exercise works on the kidneys and liver.

2) STANDING TORSO CIRCLES.
Remain seated with the feet hip width apart and a light Neck Lock. Place the hands on the hips. Rapidly rotate the torso in large circles from the hips Continue for **2 minutes and 15 seconds**.
This exercise rejuvenates the spleen and releases toxins from the liver.

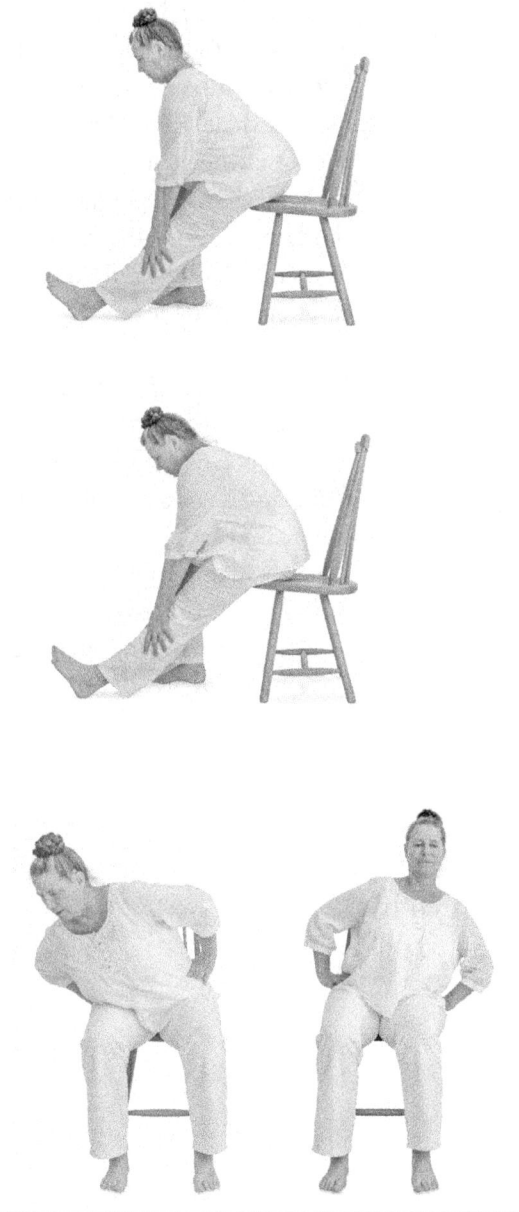

→ continue on next page

3) SPINAL TWIST VARIATION.

Sit in Easy Pose with a straight spine and a light Neck Lock. Make fists and place them in front of you, with the forearms parallel to the ground and elbows out to the sides. Twist to the left on the inhale and twist to the right on the exhale. Keep the elbows up and let the neck move. Continue for **4 minutes** with a powerful breath.
This exercise works on the kidneys. The neck movement releases the blood supply to the brain.

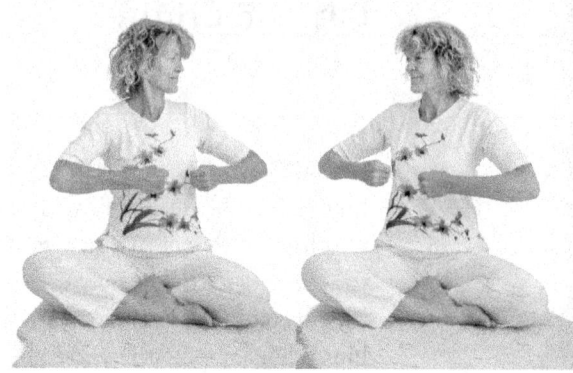

4) ONE HAND CLAPPING.

Remain in Easy Pose. Stretch the arms up at a 60-degree angle, palms facing up, fingers straight and thumbs extended out. Open and close the hands rapidly, bringing the tips of the fingers to the base of the palms. Continue for **7 minutes.**
This exercise breaks up deposits in the fingers.

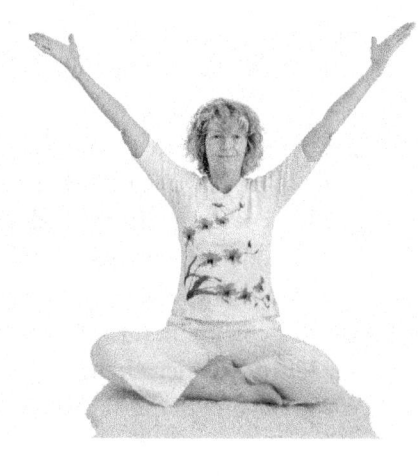

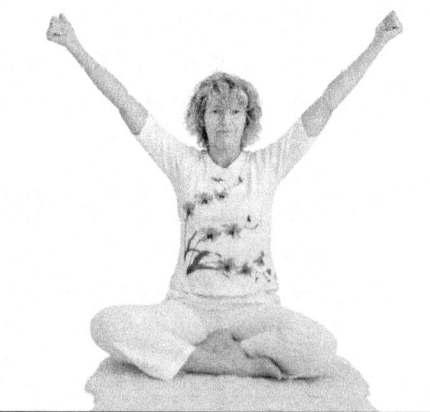

→ continue on next page

3) SPINAL TWIST VARIATION.

Remain seated. Make fists and place them in front of you, with the forearms parallel to the ground and elbows out to the sides. Twist to the left on the inhale and twist to the right on the exhale. Keep the elbows up and let the neck move. Continue for **1 minute** with a powerful breath. *This exercise works on the kidneys. The neck movement releases the blood supply to the brain.*

4) ONE HAND CLAPPING.

Remain seated. Stretch the arms up at a 60-degree angle, palms facing up, fingers straight and thumbs extended out. Open and close the hands rapidly, bringing the tips of the fingers to the base of the palms. Continue for **1 minute and 45 seconds.** *This exercise breaks up deposits in the fingers.*

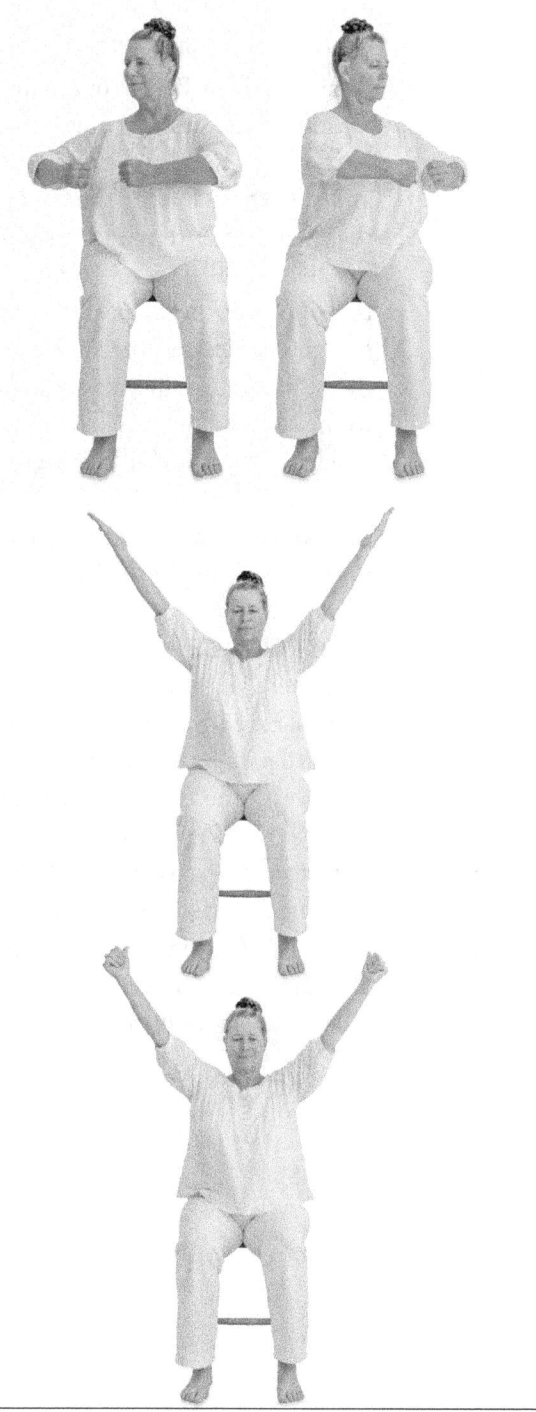

→ continue on next page

5) FISTS TO SHOULDERS.

Remain in Easy Pose. Touch the thumbs to the fleshy mound at the base of the Mercury (little) fingers and make fists, folding the fingers over the thumbs. Stretch the arms out to the sides parallel to the ground. Bend the elbows to the sides of the body, bringing the fists to the shoulders on the inhale and straighten the arms out to the sides on the exhale. Move rapidly and breathe powerfully through the "O" mouth. Continue for **6 minutes**. *This exercise removes tension from the neck and purifies the blood.*

6) FIST CIRCLES.

Remain in Easy Pose with the hands in fists. Extend the arms straight forward parallel to the ground at the level of the Heart Center, palms facing down. Rotate the fists in small outward circles. Keep the elbows straight, fists tight and move from the wrists. Continue for **2 minutes**. *This exercise adjusts the muscles under the breasts.*

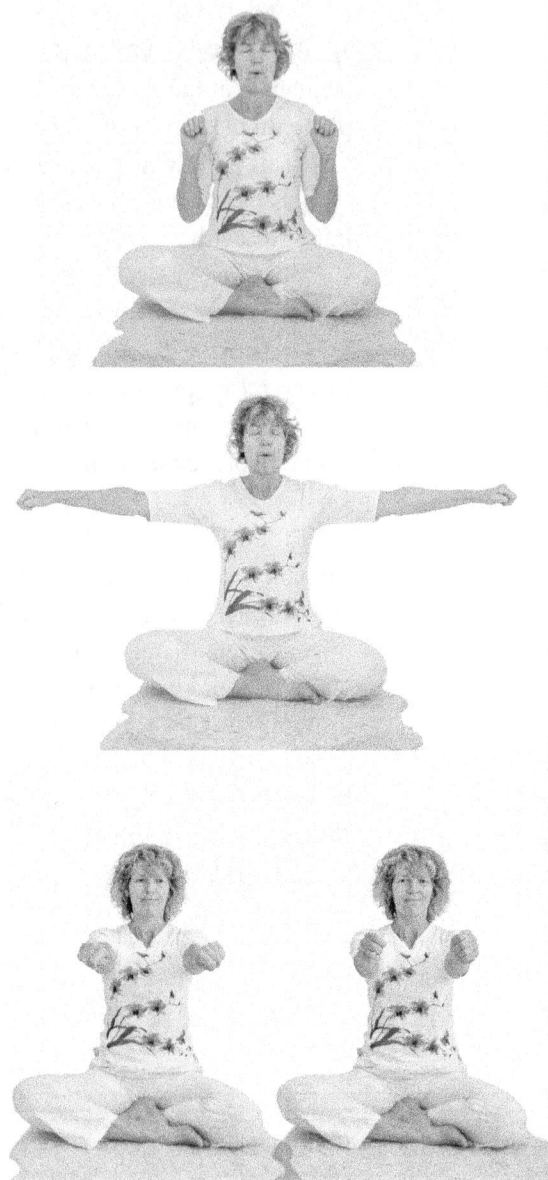

→ continue on next page

5) FISTS TO SHOULDERS.
Remain seated. Touch the thumbs to the fleshy mound at the base of the Mercury (little) fingers and make fists, folding the fingers over the thumbs. Stretch the arms out to the sides parallel to the ground. Bend the elbows to the sides of the body, bringing the fists to the shoulders on the inhale and straighten the arms out to the sides on the exhale. Move rapidly and breathe powerfully through the "O" mouth. Continue for **1 ½ minutes**. *This exercise removes tension from the neck and purifies the blood.*

6) FIST CIRCLES.
Remain seated with the hands in fists. Extend the arms straight forward parallel to the ground at the level of the Heart Center. Rotate the fists in small outward circles. Keep the elbows straight, the fists tight and move from the wrists. Continue for **1 minute**. *This exercise adjusts the muscles under the breasts.*

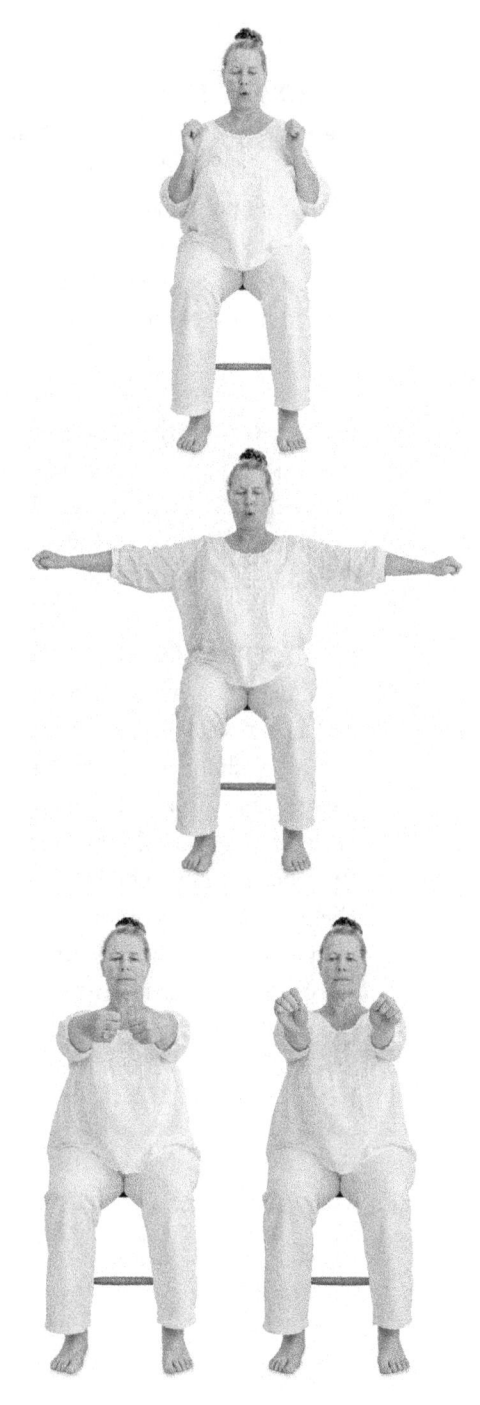

→ continue on next page

7) CROW POSE[1].

Stand with the feet hip-width apart, knees, ankles, and feet are closer to parallel alignment. Apply Root Lock and Neck Lock to keep the spine elongated. Squat down, keeping the spine as perpendicular to the ground as possible. Make fists of the hands, bend the elbows and place the fists at the sides of the neck, just above the shoulders. Inhale as you stand up and exhale as you squat down into a Crow Pose. The hands stay in place throughout the movement. Continue for **3 minutes**.

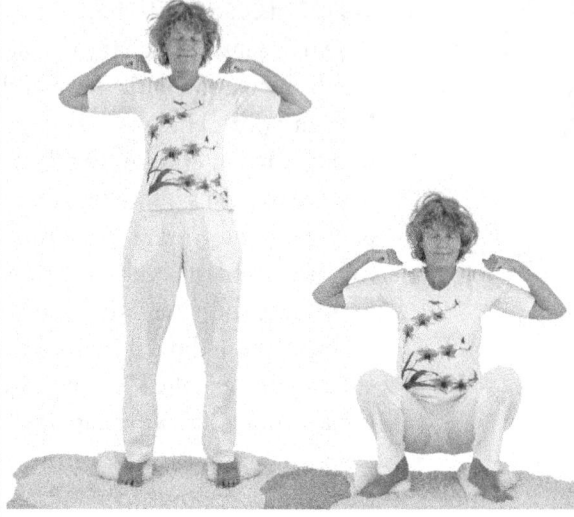

8) SITALI PRANAYAM.

Sit in Easy Pose with a straight spine and a light Neck Lock. Curl the tongue into a "U" shape and extend it slightly past the lips[2]. Inhale deeply through the curled tongue, exhale through the nose. Breathe long and deep for **4-5 minutes**. Then continue this breath in rhythm with healing music for **2 minutes**. (In the original class, a recording of "Dukh Bhanjan" was played[3].)

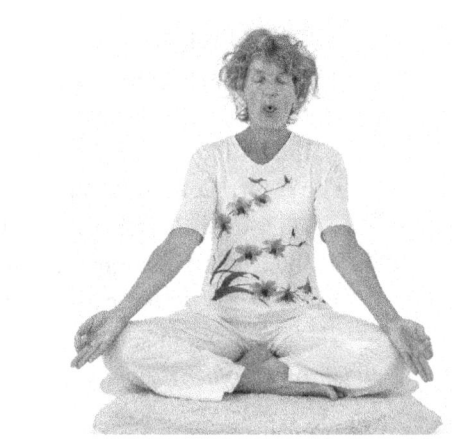

---

1 Authors' Note: If necessary, do the exercise standing behind a chair for more balance. For support, you can place a block or rolled-up blanket under your heels.
2 Authors' Note: It is genetically determined if you can curl your tongue this way or not. If you don't manage, stick out your tongue a bit and breathe through the narrow opening over your protruding tongue. Exhale slowly and deeply through the nose.
3 The shabad "Dukh Bhajan" is a sacred Sikh song in praise of the healing water that surrounds the Golden Temple. The Golden Temple represents a place of

→ continue on next page

7) CROW POSE.

Remain seated with the hands in fists. Bend the elbows and place the fists at the sides of the neck, just above the shoulders. Inhale and lift one knee as high as possible. Exhale and lower the knee again. Repeat with the other leg. The hands stay in place throughout the movement. Continue the alternate movement for **45 seconds**.

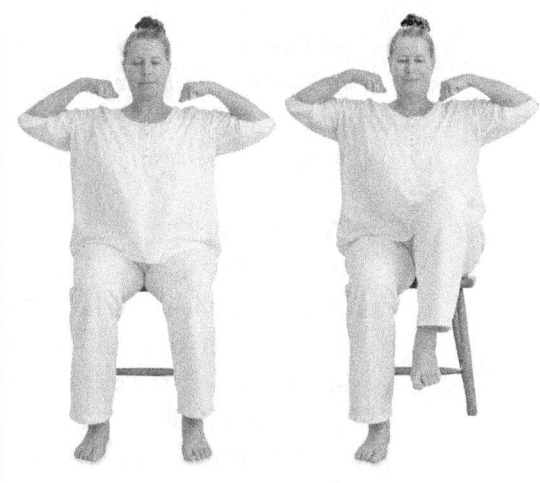

8) SITALI PRANAYAM.

Remain seated. Curl the tongue into a "U" shape and extend it slightly past the lips. Inhale deeply through the curled tongue, exhale through the nose[1]. Breathe long and deep for **1 minute**. Then continue this breath in rhythm with healing music for **1 minute**. (In the original class, a recording of "Dukh Bhanjan" was played[2].) *Sitali Pranayam is effective against anger, bad moods and temperament. If your mouth becomes bitter, it*

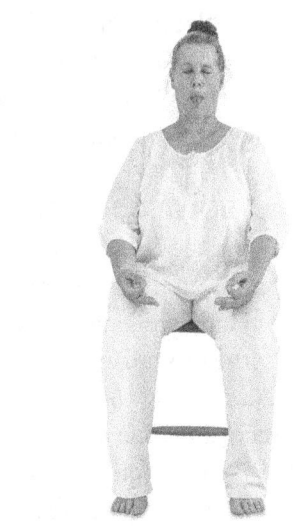

---

1 Authors' Note: It is genetically determined if you can curl your tongue this way or not. If you don't manage, stick out your tongue a bit and breathe through the narrow opening over your protruding tongue. Exhale slowly and deeply through the nose.
2 The shabad "Dukh Bhajan" is a sacred Sikh song in praise of the healing water that surrounds the Golden Temple. The Golden Temple represents a place of prayer and healing for many. It is a beautiful temple in Amritsar, India, that is the most sacred shrine of the Sikhs. It is an open house of worship for all people and is surrounded on all sides by a tank of water.

→ continue on next page

Sitali Pranayam is effective against anger, bad moods and temperament. If your mouth becomes bitter, it means you are releasing toxins.

9) SITTING DANCE.

Remain in Easy Pose and raise the arms relaxed above the head. Close the eyes and rhythmically move your arms and body to the music, without thinking. Keep the arms above the shoulder level and dance the upper body for **10 minutes**. (In the original class "Dukh Bhanjan" was played.) *If you can bring your body into exact rhythm with the music, you can go into a state of ecstasy.*

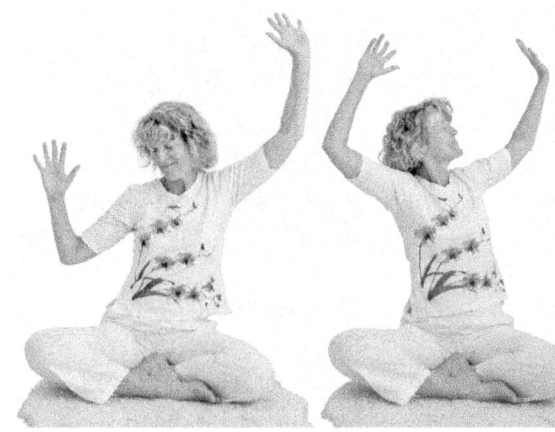

10) BOWING JAAP SAHIB.

Sit on the heels in Rock Pose, with hands on thighs. Listen to a recording of Jaap Sahib and bring the forehead to the ground every time you hear "Namastang" or "Namo." Without the recording, the movement is done to 10 beats as follows: Bow down and come up in 2 counts for 4 cycles, and rest in the starting position, on counts 9 and 10. Continue for **8 minutes**.

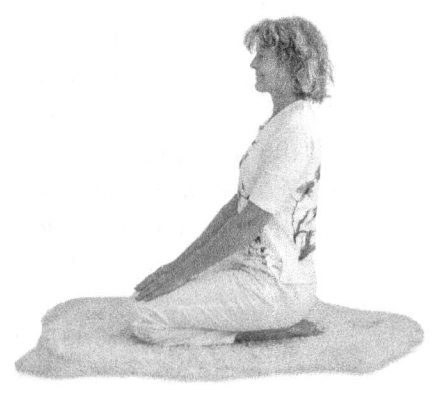

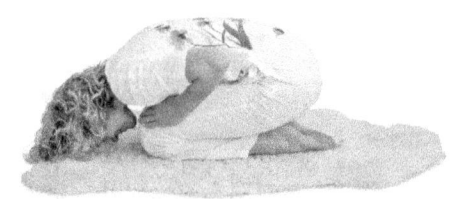

---

prayer and healing for many. It is a beautiful temple in Amritsar, India, that is the most sacred shrine of the Sikhs. It is an open house of worship for all people and is surrounded on all sides by a tank of water.

→ continue on next page

means you are releasing toxins.

9) SITTING DANCE.
Remain seated and raise the arms relaxed upward. Close the eyes and rhythmically move the arms and body to the music, without thinking. Keep the arms up and dance the upper body for **2 ½ minutes**. (In the original class, "Dukh Bhanjan" was played.)
If you can bring your body into exact rhythm with the music, you can go into a state of ecstasy.

10) BOWING JAAP SAHIB.
Remain seated with your hands on the thighs. Listen to a recording of Jaap Sahib and bring the forehead forward every time you hear "Namastang" or "Namo." Without the recording, the movement is done to 10 beats as follows: Bow down and come up in 2 counts for 4 cycles, and rest in the starting position, on counts 9 and 10. Continue for **2 minutes**.

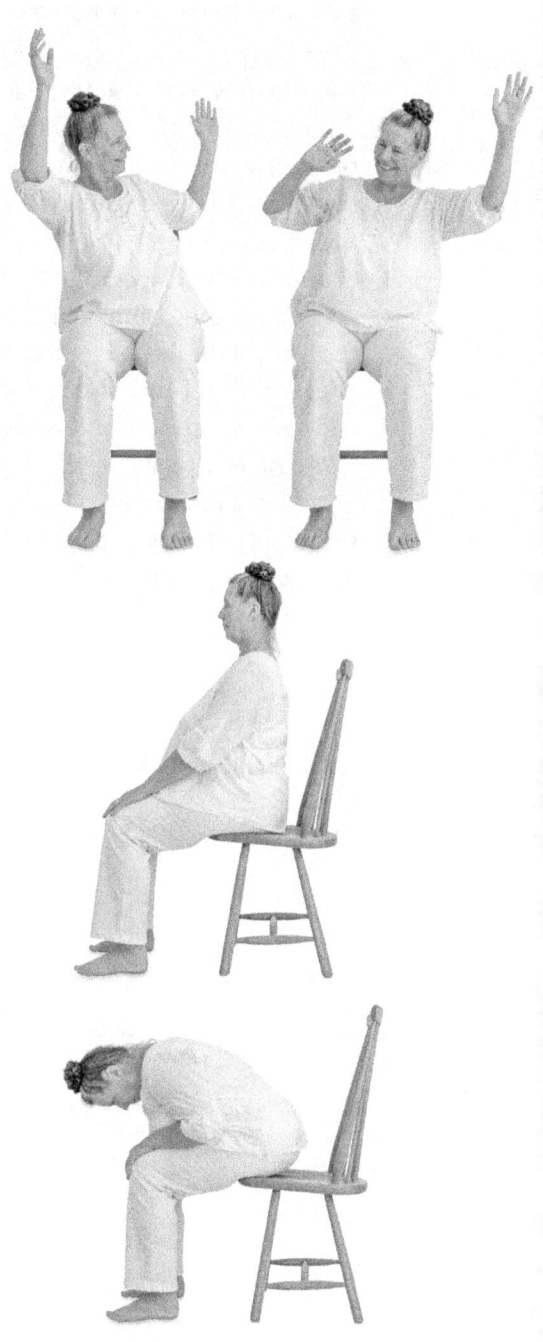

→ continue on next page

11) VENUS LOCK MEDITATION.
Sit in Easy Pose with a straight spine and a light Neck Lock. Interlace the fingers in Venus Lock, place them on the back of the head, elbows out to the sides. Apply pressure, keeping the spine straight. Close the eyes and chant out loud Jaap Sahib. Feel the vibrations going from your hands onto the back of the head. If you don't have a recording of Jaap Sahib, breathe long and deep. Continue for **8 minutes**.
Relax. Become calm. Feel that you are going to achieve God's Light in you. Totally remove any difference between yourself and God.

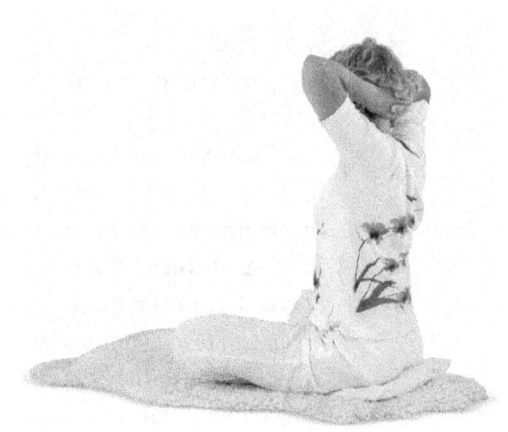

11) VENUS LOCK MEDITATION.
Remain seated with a light Neck Lock. Interlace the fingers in Venus Lock behind the head, elbows to the sides while keeping the spine straight. Close the eyes and chant out loud the Jaap Sahib. Feel the vibrations from your hands onto the back of your head. If you don't have a recording of the Jaap Sahib, breathe long and deep. Continue for **2 minutes**. *Relax. Become calm. Feel that you are going to achieve God's Light in you. Totally remove any difference between yourself and God.*

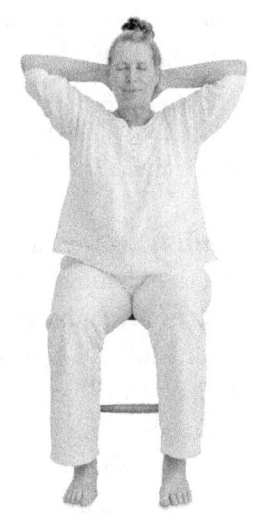

1.3 Pran Bandha Mantra
Originally published in the Aquarian Teacher Yoga Manual

Sit in Easy Pose with a straight spine and a light Neck Lock.

Mudra: Let the hands rest in the lap, right hand on the left or just sit with both hands on the knees in Gyan Mudra. Become completely still, physically and mentally, like a calm ocean. Listen to the chant for a minute. Feel its rhythm in every cell. Then chant the mantra below.

Eye Focus: Third Eye Point, at the screen of the forehead. Roll the eyes up slightly.

Mantra: PAVAN PAVAN PAVAN PAVAN, PAR PARAA, PAVAN GUROO, PAVAN GUROO, WHAA-HAY GUROO, WHAA-HAY GUROO PAVAN GUROO[1]

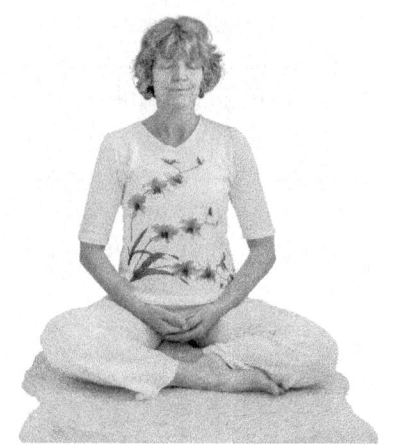

Time: 11-31 minutes.

---

1 Authors' Note: "Pavan" means air, wind, breath, praana. Wherever there is praana, there is a potential to move, change. "Par" is finite, visible, and frivolous. "Para" is past the finite, invisible, untouchable, infinite.

→ continue on next page

ON THE CHAIR

Sit comfortably in a chair with the weight of both feet resting evenly on the ground, with a straight spine and a light Neck Lock.

Practice as described on the side.

Time: Continue for at least **5 ½ minutes**.

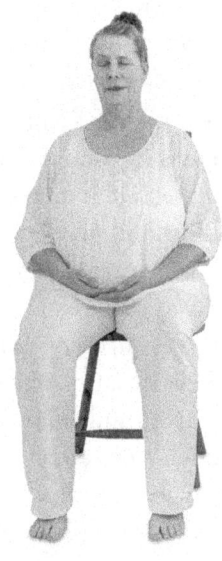

Comments: Pran Bandha Mantra means that mantra that collects, binds, and commands the life force or praana. In our usual non-liberated state, we are controlled by our attachments. We become attached to our finite identity, or to time, space, and intensity of emotion or experience. This mantra takes you beyond those finite attachments. It opens the door to another dimension of the Self. It merges you into the unlimited sea of praana and life. This mantra forges a link between you as a finite magnetic field and the universal, creative magnetic field of energy that we call consciousness. Prayers and mental desires become much more effective. This meditation can give you the capacity to embody a divine personality and to become creative and fearless.

CHAPTER 2
Hard Decisions
—

Consciously ask your intuition to show you the path.
Consciously ask your courage to face the calamity.
Ask your grace to face the insecurity.
Ask your breath of life to face depression.
Rise, rise and excel.
— YOGI BHAJAN, JUNE 30, 1994

This chapter focuses on the life theme of preparing yourself for making hard decisions. Begin by discovering what patterns lie underneath decision-making, and how to find the inner resources to make these difficult decisions. Often emotions can block the ability to move forward, and they can play tricks on you; for example, how anger or blame can divert your energy in the wrong direction, or how fear can paralyze you. Perhaps you have an internal conflict that you experience when faced with decision-making. Or you can do shadow work and learn how to bring it to light. You can work on forgiveness as a resource, as it benefits both you and the other person. Finally, you can ease your way forward with decision-making by being flexible and building a solid foundation to make decisions from this supporting place.

The yoga and meditation in this chapter help you to become more aware of how to make difficult decisions and provide the resources that can assist you in this often challenging process. These resources are the ability to face facts, being flexible, finding your foundation, courage, forgiveness, and the ability to change.

The kriya and meditations found in this chapter have been selected to create a strong foundation and to bring out the qualities of inner knowing, healing energy, and to release inner conflicts. The *Kriya for the Back* restores your foundation, opens the heart and lungs, and relieves anxiety. The first meditation *Sending Healing Thoughts* strengthens your inner knowing, allowing you to make better decisions.

It also opens up the flow of energy in the energetic channels, which becomes a resource of healing, subtle awareness and an experience of life energy. The second meditation called *Meditation for Change* aids in feeling better about unexpected changes by surrendering to your higher self and unblocking the subconscious conflict in the mind. Find within you inner resources to make hard decisions from a strong foundation and with the healing energy that is always available to you.

2.1 Kriya for the Back
November 30, 1983

1) KNEES LIFTING.
Sit in Easy Pose with a straight spine and a light Neck Lock. Place the hands together in the center of the chest in Prayer Pose (Pranam mudra). Bring the left arm up to a 60-degree angle, palm up, as you bring both knees up as high as possible. Bring the left hand back to the original position, simultaneously clap and lower the knees. Repeat the sequence with the right arm. Alternate arms, inhaling as one arm goes up and exhaling as it goes down and lifting the knees up forcefully. Create a rhythm. Continue for **4-5 minutes**. Breathe powerfully. *This exercise is for the third vertebra and for the hip bone. Done right, it helps prevent lower back pain and develops motor coordination.*

2) HEAD TO KNEES.
Remain in Easy Pose and place the hands on the hips. Inhale deeply and exhale as you lower the head to one knee, inhale up, exhale, and lower the head to the other knee. Continue alternating sides for **3-4 minutes**.

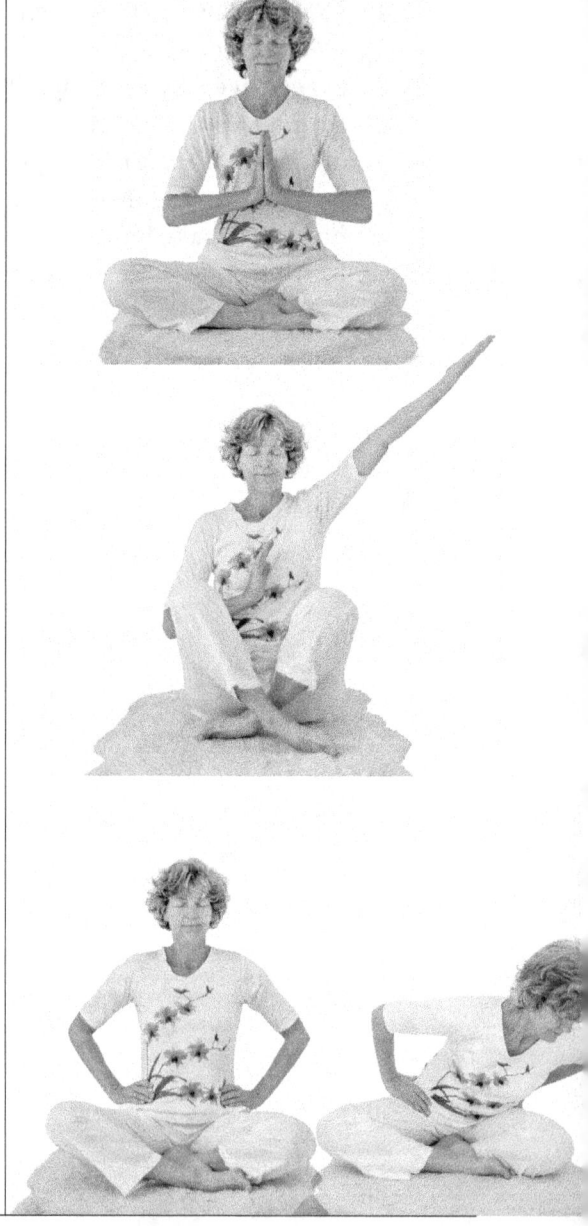

→ continue on next page

ON THE CHAIR

1) KNEES LIFTING.
Sit on the chair and cross the ankles with the knees open wide and a light Neck Lock. Place the hands together in the center of the chest in Prayer Pose (Pranam mudra). Bring the left arm up to a 60-degree angle, palm up, as you bring both knees up as high as possible. Bring the left hand back to the original position, simultaneously clap and lower the knees. Repeat the sequence with the right arm. Alternate arms, inhaling as one arm goes up and exhaling as it goes down, and lifting the knees up forcefully. Create a rhythm. Continue for **2 minutes**. Breath powerfully. *This exercise is for the third vertebra and for the hip bone. Done right, it helps prevent lower back pain and develops motor coordination.*

2) HEAD TO KNEES.
Remain seated with the feet hip-width apart and the hands on the hips. Inhale deeply and exhale as you lower the head toward one knee, inhale up, exhale and lower the head toward the other knee. Continue alternating sides for **1 ½ minutes**.

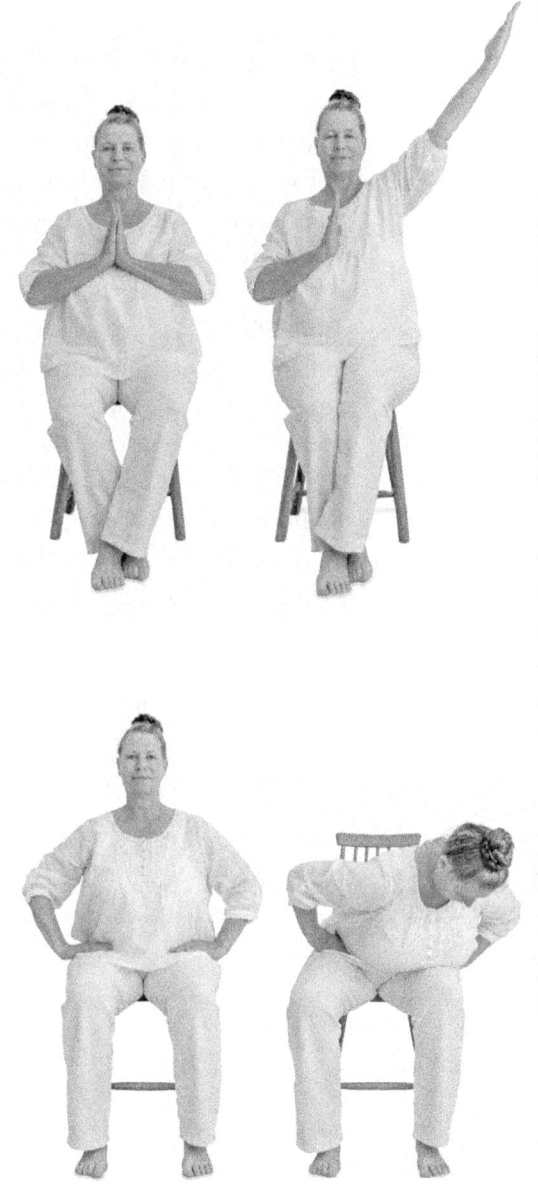

→ continue on next page

3) SPINAL FLEX.

Remain in Easy Pose. Grasp the knees firmly. Keeping the elbows straight, flex the upper spine forward and lift the chest on the inhale, and flex the upper spine backward on the exhale. The movement is at the level of the upper thoracic spine in the heart area. The head is still and remains in Neck Lock. Continue at a moderate pace for **3 minutes**. Breathe powerfully.

4) TORSO TWIST.

Remain in Easy Pose. Extend the arms out to the sides, parallel to the ground, with the forearms straight up perpendicular to the ground and palms facing forward. Twist to the left on the inhale and twist to the right on the exhale. Keep the upper arms parallel to the ground, elbows pulled back to open the chest. Initiate the movement from the Navel Point, not the arms. The head moves last. Continue for **3 minutes**. Breath powerfully.

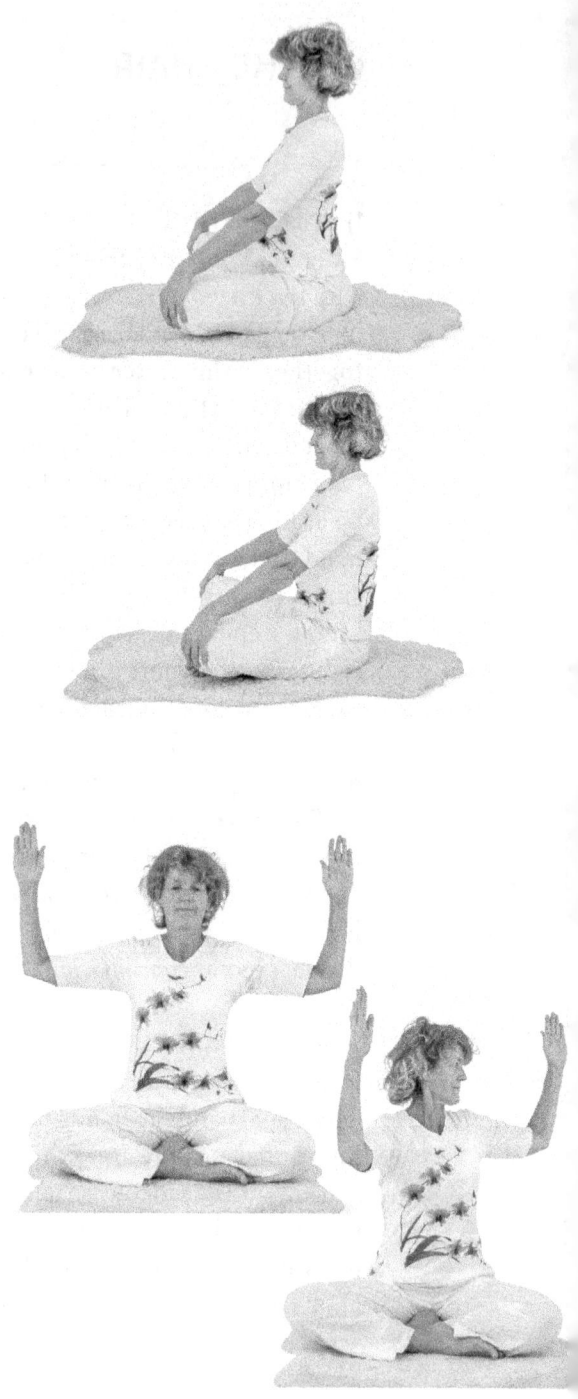

→ continue on next page

3) SPINAL FLEX.

Remain seated with the feet hip-width apart. Grasp the knees firmly. Keeping the elbows straight, flex the upper forward and lift the chest on the inhale, and flex the upper chest backward on the exhale. The movement is at the level of the upper thoracic spine in the heart area. The head is still and remains in neck Lock. Continue at a moderate pace for **1 ½ minutes**. Breath powerfully.

4) TORSO TWIST.

Remain seated. Extend the arms out to the sides, parallel to the ground, with the forearms straight up perpendicular to the ground and palms facing forward. Twist to the left on the inhale and twist to the right on the exhale. Keep the upper arms parallel to the ground, elbows pulled back to open the chest. Initiate the movement from the Navel Point, not the arms. The head moves last. Continue for **1 ½ minutes**. Breath powerfully.

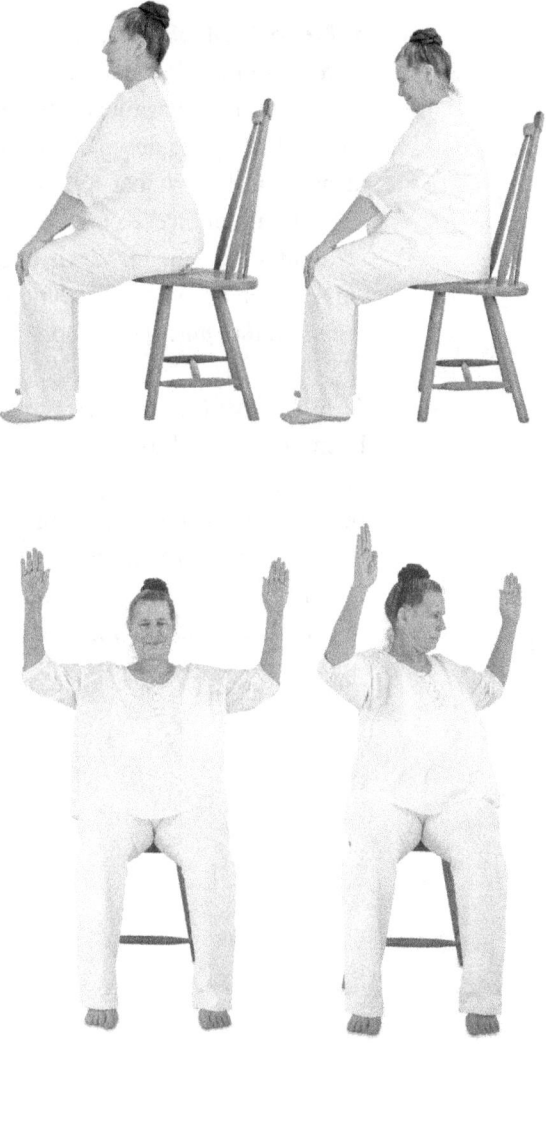

→ continue on next page

5) ARMS SWINGS (LATERAL).

Remain in Easy Pose. Extend the arms out to the sides, parallel to the ground with palms facing down. Move both arms up and down in a steady rhythm with Breath of Fire. Keep the elbows straight. Continue for **2 minutes**. *This exercise is good for the lymph glands and to purify the blood.*

6) ARMS SWINGS (FRONT).

Remain in Easy Pose. Stretch the arms straight forward parallel to the ground with the palms facing down. Once more, move both arms up and down in rhythm with Breath of Fire. Continue for **1 minute**.

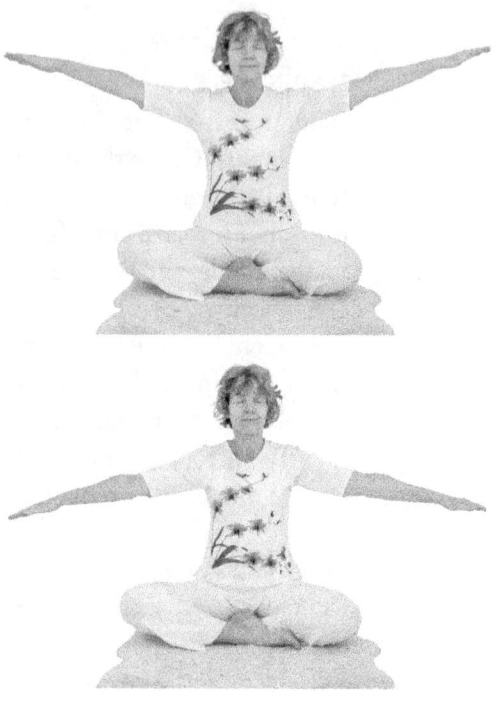
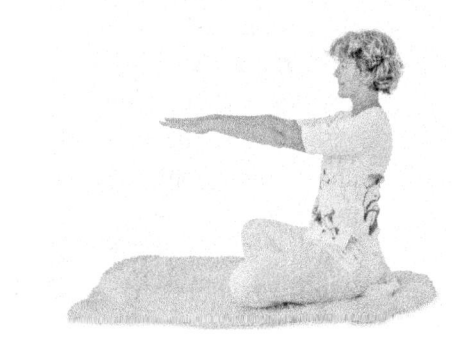

→ continue on next page

5) ARMS SWINGS (LATERAL). Remain seated. Extend the arms out to the sides, parallel to the ground with the palms facing down. Move both arms up and down in a steady rhythm with Breath of Fire. Keep the elbows straight. Continue for **1 minute**. *This exercise is good for the lymph glands and to purify the blood.*

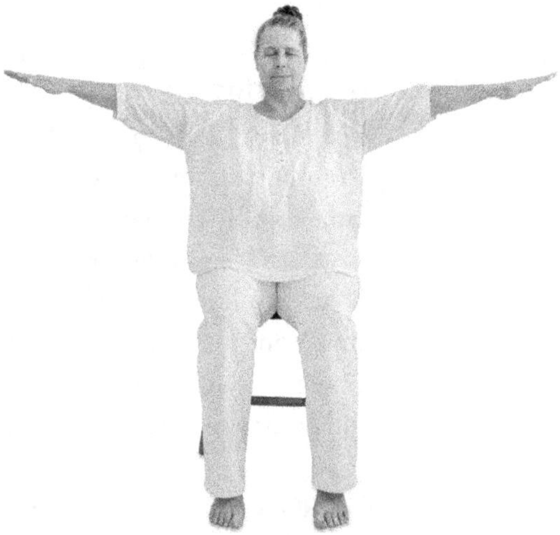

6) ARMS SWINGS (FRONT). Remain seated. Stretch the arms straight forward parallel to the ground with the palms facing down. Once more, move both arms up and down in rhythm with Breath of Fire. Continue for **1 minute**.

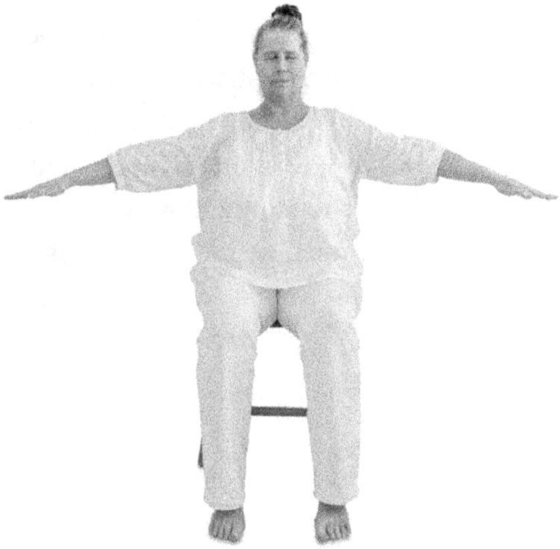

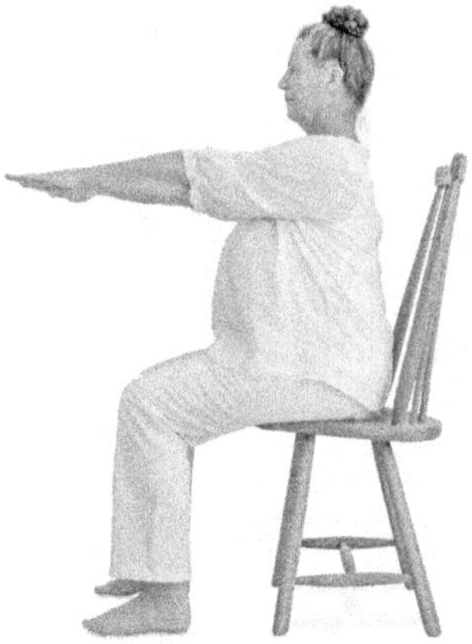

→ continue on next page

7) ARM CIRCLES.

Remain in Easy Pose with the arms stretched forward. Move both arms rapidly from front to back in large circles as if you were doing a backstroke. Chant **HAR** in a monotone synchronized with the movement. Keep the arms straight and continue for **30 seconds**.

8) CROW POSE VARIATION[1].

Squat in Crow Pose with the feet shoulder-width apart, toes facing slightly out, and hands on the hips. Stand up and squat down as you chant **HAR** in a monotone synchronized with the movement. Continue for **2 minutes**.

This exercise is not recommended for pregnant women.

---

[1] Authors' Note: If necessary, do the exercise standing behind a chair for more balance. For support, you can place a block or rolled-up blanket under your heels.

7) ARM CIRCLES.
Remain seated with the arms stretched forward. Move both arms rapidly from front to back in large circles as if you were doing a backstroke. Chant **HAR** in a monotone synchronized with the movement. Keep the arms straight and continue for **30 seconds**.

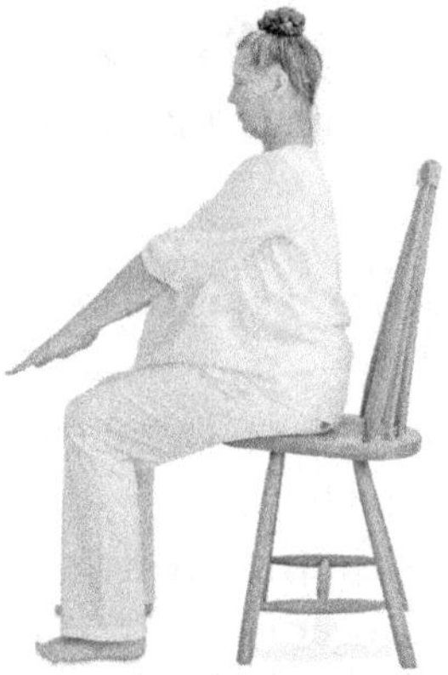

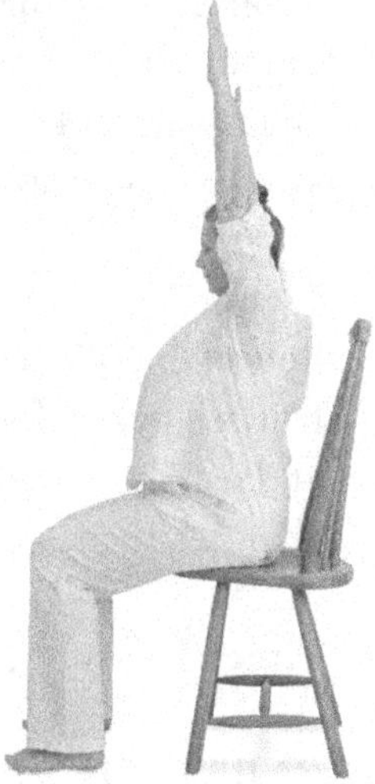

8) CROW POSE VARIATION.
Remain seated and place the hands on the hips. Lift one knee while inhaling and put your foot back on the ground while exhaling. Chant **HAR** in a monotone synchronized with the movement. Continue for **1 minute**. *This exercise is not recommended for pregnant women.*

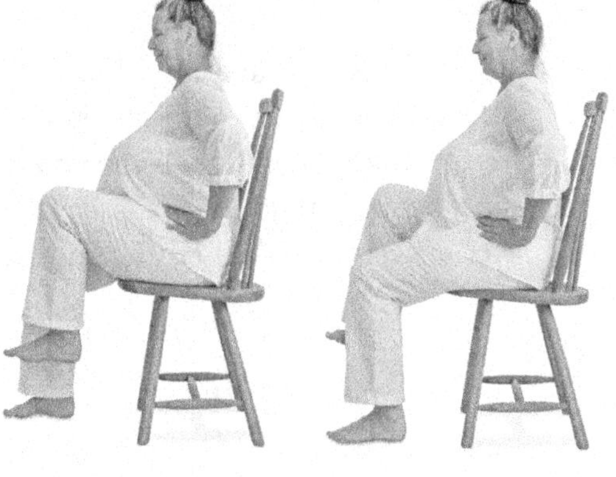

2.2 Sending Healing Thoughts Meditation
November 20, 1970

WARM UP
Sit in Easy Pose with a straight spine and a light Neck Lock.

Mudra: Briefly rub the hands together. Raise them facing each other no more than **6 inches (15 cm)** apart in front of the chest at Heart Center level. Keep the hands straight and fingers pointing upward.

Mental Focus: Concentrate on the flow of energy between the palms, from right to left and left to right, and feel the central spinal energy channel, the silver cord (*sushumna*).

Time: Continue for **3-5 minutes**.

PART ONE
Sit in Easy Pose with a straight spine and a light Neck Lock.

Mudra: Place the palms together at the center of the chest in Prayer Pose. Press the hands firmly together and press the total weight of the body against them.

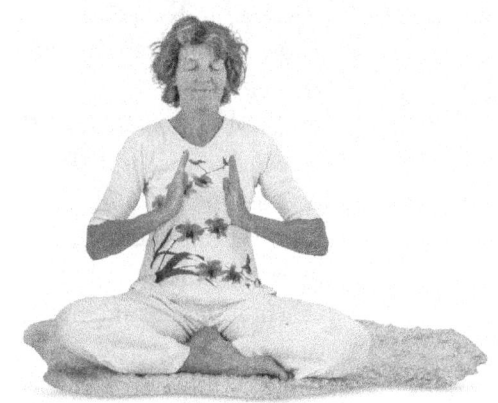

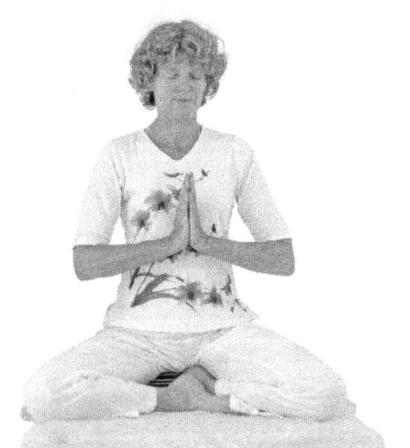

→ continue on next page

ON THE CHAIR

Sit comfortably in a chair with the weight of both feet resting evenly on the ground, with a straight spine and a light Neck Lock.

Practice as described on the side.

WARM-UP
Time: Start with **1 minute** and build up to **3 minutes**.

PART ONE
a) Start with **1 minute** and build up to **3 minutes**.
b) Start with **3 minutes** and build up to **6 minutes**.

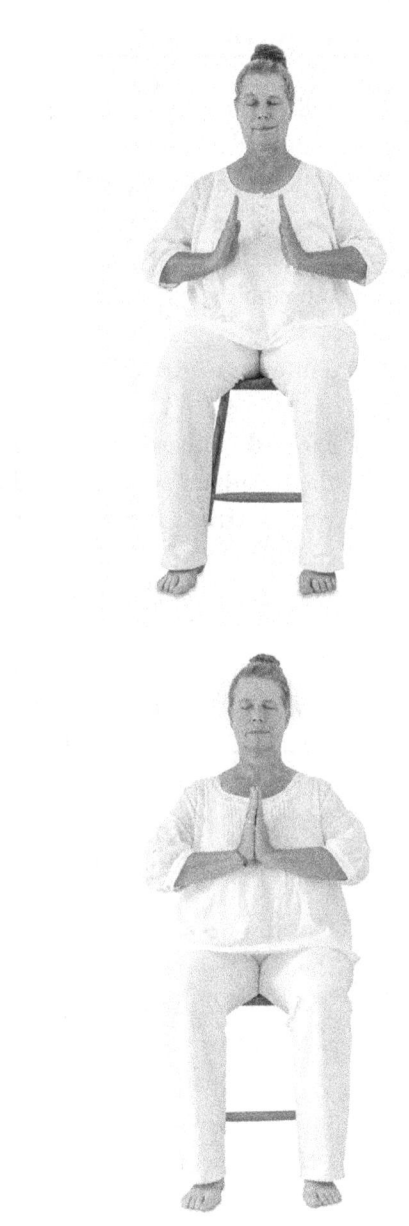

a) Mental Focus: Concentrate and open the Heart Center. Fill it with love; eliminate fear and anger.

Time: 3 minutes.

b) Mental Focus: Recognize the beautiful magnetic field around you. Feel and vibrate the energy you created and project it. Imagine you are on the top of a mountain sending out rippling waves of healing energy.

Time: 6 minutes.

To End: Inhale deeply, suspend the breath for **10-15 seconds**, fill your heart with love and project the life force, praana to those who need it. Exhale. Repeat this breath **1 more time**. Inhale deeply, suspend the breath for up to **30 seconds** and concentrate this breath in the Heart Center and feel the energy flowing through your hands out to those in need. Exhale. Repeat this breath **2 more times**. Relax.

Comments: With sincere practice, the channels will open enabling you to send this healing energy to anyone that you imagine. With permission, this healing projection can be sent to someone you love.

2.3 Meditation for Change
October 22, 1971

Sit in Easy Pose with a straight spine and a light Neck Lock.

Mudra: Bring the hands in front or the Heart Center. Make fists of the hands with the thumbs extended. The hands touch lightly in two places only: the knuckles of the Saturn (middle) fingers and the pads of the thumbs. The thumbs point toward the body. Hold this position and feel the energy between the thumbs and knuckles.

Breath: Long Deep Breathing.

Time: **31 minutes**.

To End: Inhale deeply and relax for **5 minutes**.

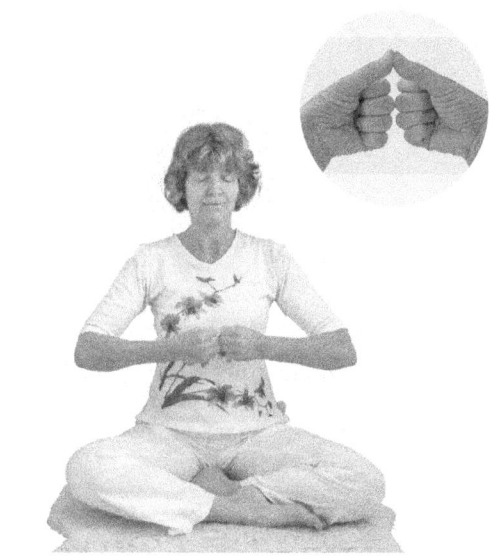

Comments: After practicing and mastering **31 minutes**, you may add another **31 minutes** after the rest period. Change is a universal principle of life. However, the attachment to the ego is resistant to change. This creates a constant hassle in the mind between perceived reality from the ego and potential reality. To be happy in life's changes, you must surrender yourself to your higher Self. Practicing this meditation daily can change your ego identification and unblock the subconscious conflict in the mind.

ON THE CHAIR

Sit on the chair with the feet hip-width apart and flat on the ground, with a straight spine and a light Neck Lock.

Practice as described on the side.

Time: Continue for **3 minutes**. Then relax for **2 minutes** and repeat the meditation for **3 more minutes**.

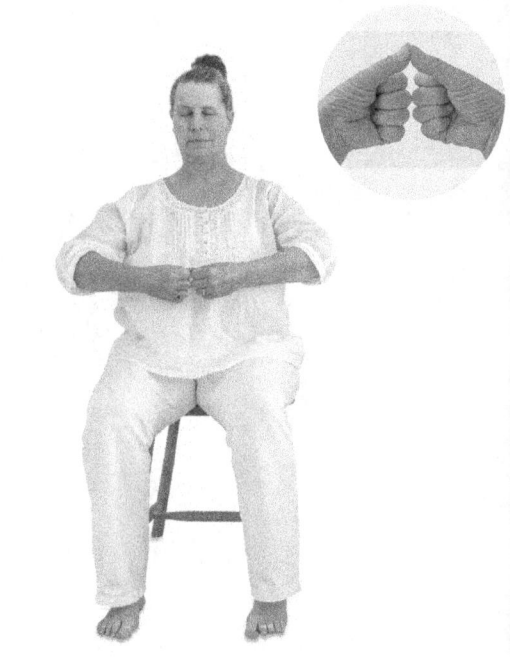

CHAPTER 3
Loss and Grief

—

The greatest art is to sit, and wait, and let it come.
— YOGI BHAJAN, JANUARY 14, 1985

In this chapter you will work on the life theme of coming to terms with loss, mourning and letting go. You will also discover the self-care that is needed in times of misplacement. It is important to become aware of what you need during a period of loss or mourning, taking your own pace and natural rhythm into account. Understand that everyone goes through this process in their own unique way. Yoga practice, breathing exercises and meditation are all helpful resources for self-care. The selected kriya and meditations can assist you in processing a loss. If you feel like you want to go further, you can also choose different breathing exercises, meditations or kriyas from this book if necessary. It is up to you to sense what resources can help you the most at this moment.

To console and inspire you in this chapter, we share below a quote about love from the author Courtney A. Walsh, from her book *Dear Human: A Manifesto of Love, Invitation and Invocation to Humanity*. She reminds us that human experience is impermanent and that we are here to experience life as it is, with its flaws and messiness but also with its grace, divinity and beauty.

> *"Dear Human, You've got it all wrong. You didn't come here to master unconditional love. This is where you came from and where you'll return. You came here to learn personal love. Universal love. Messy love. Sweaty love. Crazy love. Broken love. Whole love. Infused with divinity. Lived through the grace of stumbling. Demonstrated through the beauty of... messing up. Often. You didn't come here to be perfect. You already are. You came here to be gorgeously human. Flawed and fabulous. And rising again into remembering. But unconditional love? Stop telling that story. Love, in truth, doesn't need*

> *any adjectives. It doesn't require modifiers. It doesn't require the condition of perfection. It only asks you to show up. And do your best. That you stay present and feel fully. That you shine and fly and laugh and cry and hurt and heal and fall and get back up and play and work and live and die as YOU. It's enough. It's plenty.[1]"*

The kriya and meditations selected for this chapter are centered on self-care practices, cooling pranayama and slow-moving yoga to calm the body, mind and nervous system, and at last, finding the inner connection with the Self. The first meditation is a pranayama or breath-focused meditation and is called *The Meditation to Prevent Freaking Out*. It changes your energy, allowing you to cool down and relax. The *Evening Kriya* relaxes the body and prepares you for sleep, as it is done in a very slow and relaxing manner. The second meditation called *Meditation to Remove Fear of the Future* aids in letting go of fear of the future through connecting the Self at the Heart Center. Find solace in practicing gentle self-care, in slowing down and resting in the space of the heart.

---

1 Courtney A. Walsh. Dear Human: A Manifesto of Love, Invitation and Invocation to Humanity. (Scotland: Findhorn Press, 2016), p. 14.

3.1 Meditation to Prevent Freaking Out
June 7, 1976

Sit in Easy Pose with a straight spine and a light Neck Lock.

Mudra: Interlace your fingers with your right thumb on top. Place your hands at the center of your diaphragm line, touching your body. Maintain the shoulders completely relaxed. You should have pressure at your hands but none at your shoulders.

Eye Focus: Closed.

Breath: Concentrate on your breath at the Tip of the Nose. Be aware of which nostril you are breathing. Within 3 minutes you should know. Then change it. If you are breathing primarily through your left nostril, consciously change to your right nostril.

Time: 11-31 minutes.

Comments: The ability to be aware of and consciously change which nostril is active is a simple helpful practice that even a young child can learn. Switching the dominant nostril breath can change your mental state. For example, if you are irritated or depressed, try breathing through the right nostril and see what happens.

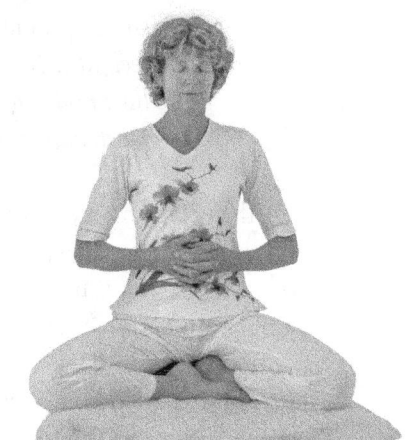

ON THE CHAIR

Sit on the chair with the feet hip-width apart and flat on the ground, with a straight spine and a light Neck Lock.

Practice as described on the side.

Time: Start with **3 minutes** and gradually build up to **11 minutes**.

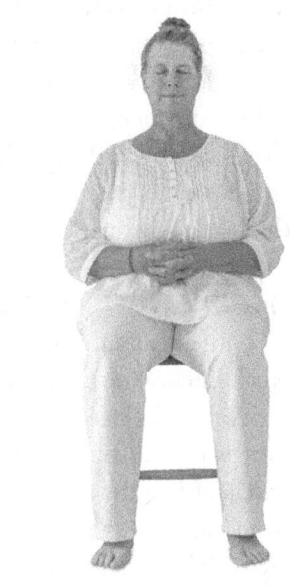

3.2 Evening Kriya
Originally published in The Aquarian Times, June 2007

1) LOWER SPINE MASSAGE.
Lie on the back and draw both knees to the chest. Keep the head on the ground and wrap the arms around the legs just below the knees. Pull the knees to the chest and then release. Create a slow rhythm while consciously relaxing the back. Continue for **2 minutes**.

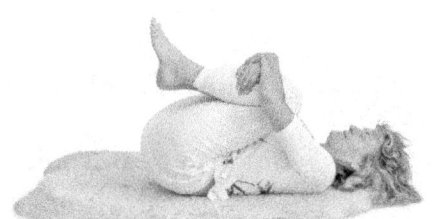

2) LIFE NERVE STRETCH (LEFT & RIGHT).
Sit with a straight spine and a light Neck Lock. Stretch the left leg straight forward and place the sole of the right foot against the inner left thigh. Inhale and lengthen the spine. Exhale, bend from the hips, and reach over the left leg with both hands. Grasp the left foot or as far down as possible. Keep the spine and leg straight and the sternum lifted with a light Neck Lock. Relax in this position with slow, deep breathing through the nose. Continue for **1 ½ minutes**. Switch legs and repeat on the right side. Continue for **1 ½ minutes**.

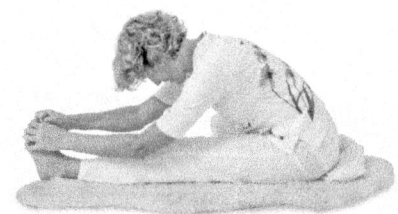

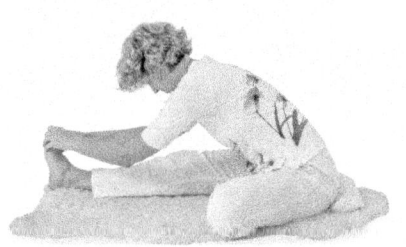

→ continue on next page

ON THE CHAIR

1) LOWER SPINE MASSAGE.
Sit on the chair with the feet hip-width apart flat on the ground and a light Neck Lock. Slide a bit forward on the seat of the chair, and stretch the back a bit. Raise the left leg and grasp the left shin. Gently pull your left leg toward your chest and then slowly put the foot down on the ground. Alternate raising the legs in a slow and easy rhythm, while you consciously relax the lower back. Continue for **1 minute**.

2) LIFE NERVE STRETCH (LEFT & RIGHT).
Remain seated with your right foot firmly on the ground and stretch your left leg forward. Inhale and lengthen the spine. Exhale, bend from the hips, and reach over the left leg with both hands. Grasp the leg as far down as possible – the ankle, calf or thigh. Keep the spine and leg straight, and the sternum lifted with a light Neck Lock. Relax in this position with slow, deep breathing through the nose. Continue for **45 seconds**. Switch legs stretching on the right side. Continue for **45 seconds**.

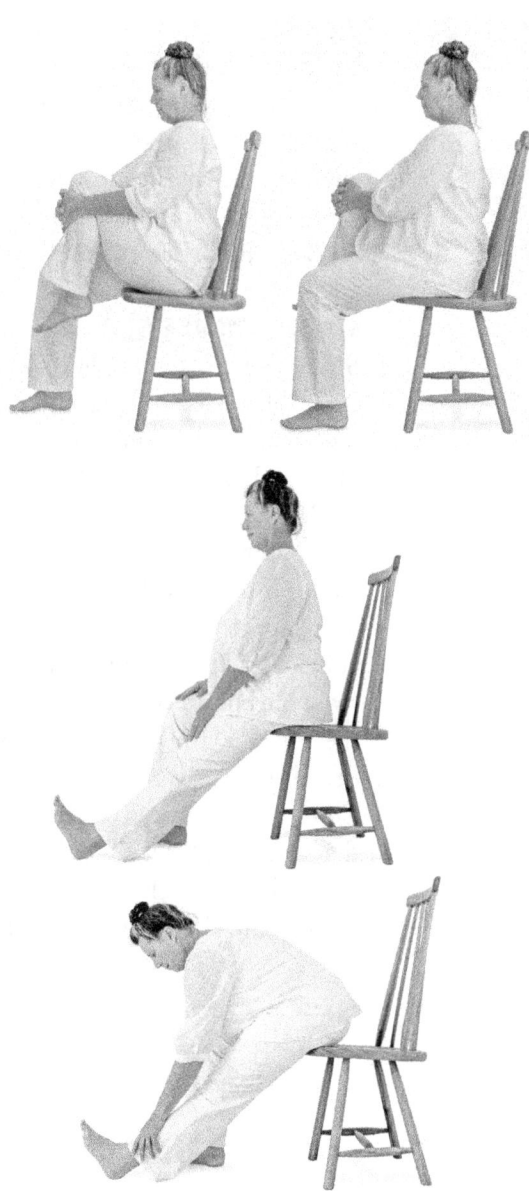

→ continue on next page

3) CAMEL RIDE.

Sit in Easy Pose with a straight spine and a light Neck Lock. Grasp the shins or ankles with the hands. Tilt the pelvis forward on the inhale and backward on the exhale. Only the pelvis and lower spine move. The rib cage, shoulders, and head are still and remain over the hips. The motion is fluid and continuous. Continue for **2 minutes**. Breathe powerfully.

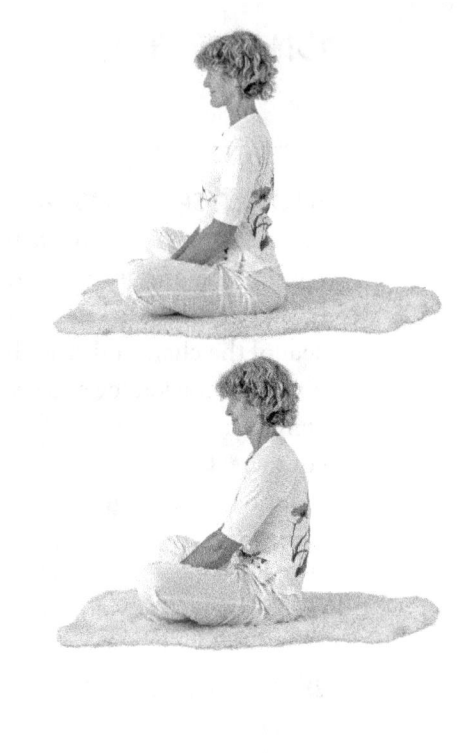

4) HALF-SPINAL TWIST.

Stretch your legs straight forward. Bend the left leg and place the left foot flat on the ground, just outside of the right knee. Bring the left hand on the ground behind you on the left side. Wrap the right arm around the left leg just below the knee. Inhale and lengthen the spine, keep the chin level to the ground, exhale and twist the body as far as possible to the left. Hold the position with slow, deep breathing through the nose. Continue for **1 minute**, then reverse the posture, so the left leg is straight forward, the right leg bent, and twist to the right. Continue for **1 minute**.

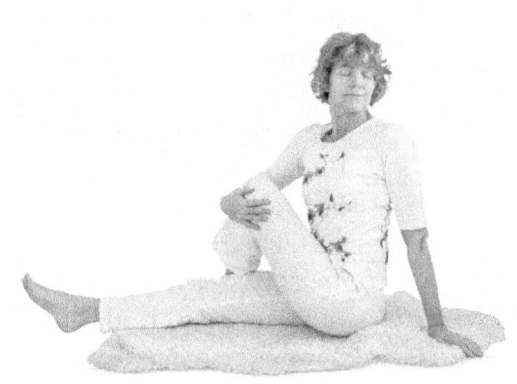

→ continue on next page

3) CAMEL RIDE.

Remain seated with the hands on the upper thighs at the crease of the hips. Tilt the pelvis forward on the inhale and backward on the exhale. Only the pelvis and lower spine move. The rib cage, shoulders and head are still and remain over the hips. The motion is fluid and continuous. Continue for **1 minute**. Breathe powerfully.

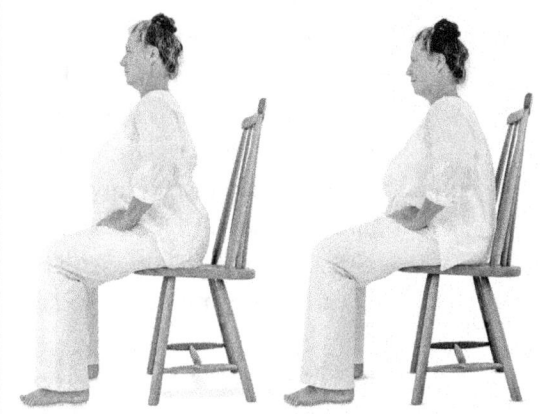

4) HALF SPINAL TWIST.

Remain seated with the left foot firmly on the ground and right leg stretched forward. Grasp the left side of the seat with your left hand or place it behind you on the chair. Place your right hand on your left thigh. Lengthen your spine and gently twist the body to the left. Hold this position with slow, deep breathing through the nose. Continue for **1 minute**. Then switch sides: stretch your left leg and grasp the right side of the seat with your right hand or place it behind you on the chair. Place your left hand on your right thigh. Lengthen the spine, and gently twist the body to the right. Hold this position with Long Deep Breathing. Continue for **1 minute**.

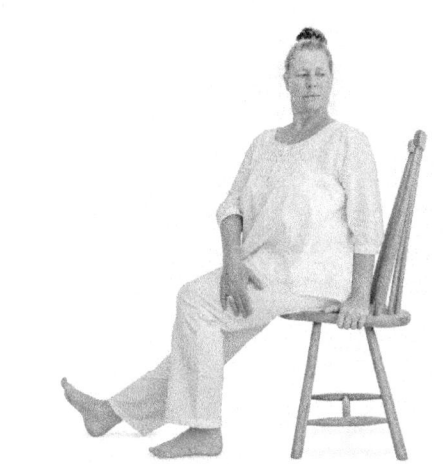

→ continue on next page

5) COW POSE.

Come onto your hands and knees with knees directly under the hips and arms straight, palms flat on the ground directly under the shoulders. Arch the spine downward, lowering the abdomen and lifting the sternum and chin. Hold the position with Long Deep Breathing. Continue for **45 seconds**.

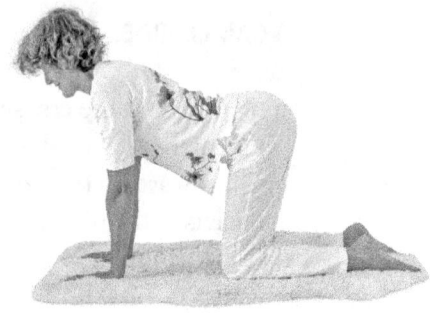

6) CAT POSE.

Remain on your hands and knees, round the spine up toward the ceiling, and bring the chin toward the chest. Hold the position with Long Deep Breathing. Continue for **45 seconds**.

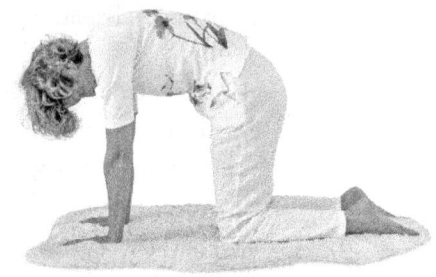

7) CAT COW.

Inhale into Cow Pose and exhale into Cat Pose. The motion is fluid and relaxed. Continue for **1 minute**.

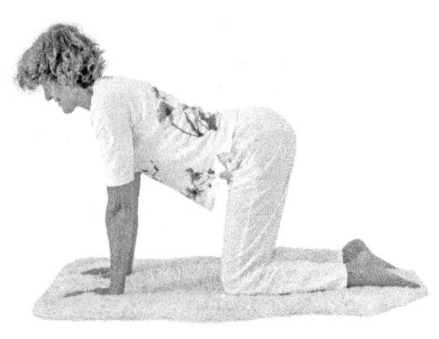

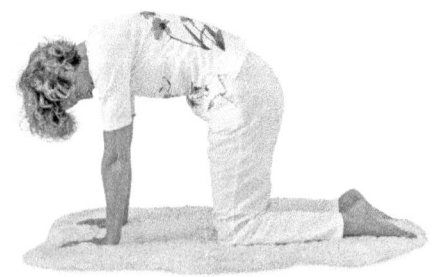

→ continue on next page

5) COW POSE.
Remain seated with feet hip-width apart and the hands on the thighs. Gently tilt the pelvis forward, arching the back and opening your chest; lift the chin slightly. Stay in this posture with Long Deep Breathing. Continue for **45 seconds**.

6) CAT POSE.
Remain seated with the feet hip-width apart and the hands on the thighs. Gently tilt the pelvis backward and draw the stomach inward, arching the back; bring the chin toward your chest. Stay in this posture with a Long Deep Breathing. Continue for **45 seconds**.

7) CAT COW.
Remain seated with the feet hip-width apart and the hands on the thighs. Inhale into Cow Pose and exhale into Cat Pose. The motion is fluid and relaxed. Continue for **1 minute**.

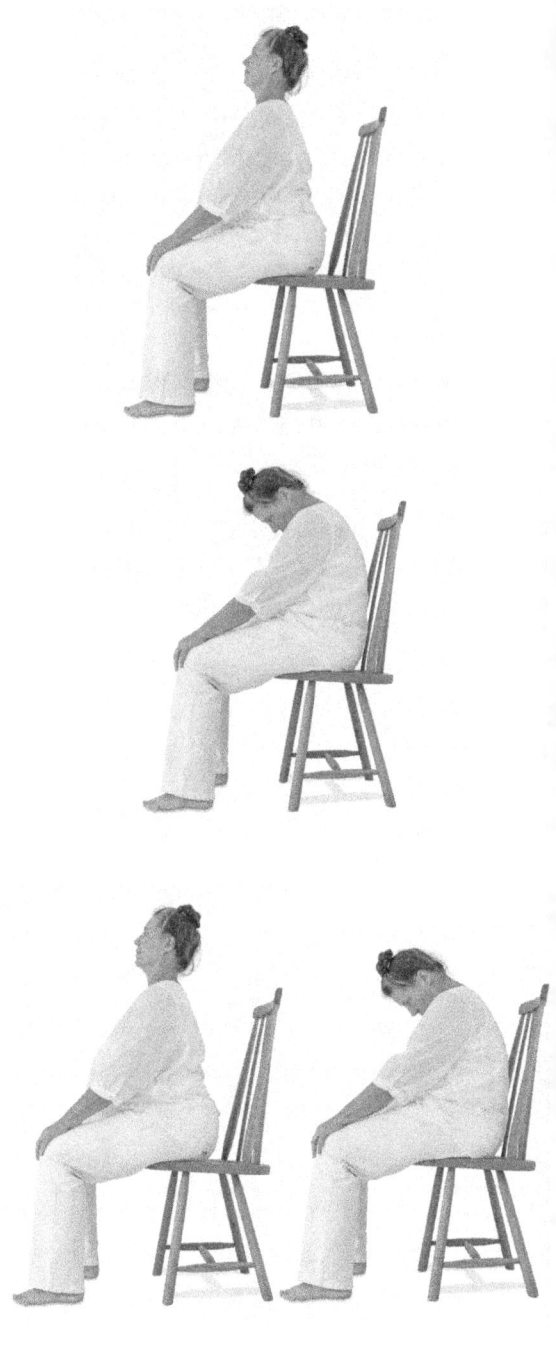

→ continue on next page

8) BABY POSE VARIATION.

Sit on your heels in Rock Pose and bring the forehead to the ground. Stretch the arms straight forward with the palms flat against the ground. Breathe naturally and relax for **45 seconds**.

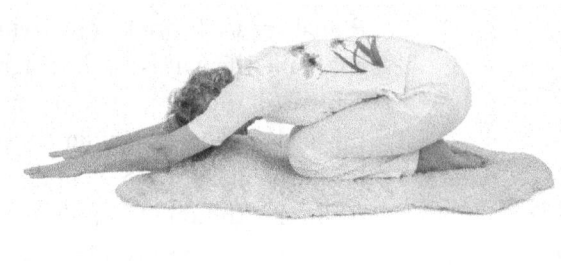

9) SHOULDER ROLLS.

Sit in Easy Pose with the hands on the knees. Roll the shoulders forward in large circles for **30 seconds**. Reverse the direction and roll the shoulders backward in large circles for another **30 seconds**. Breathe normally. Relax.

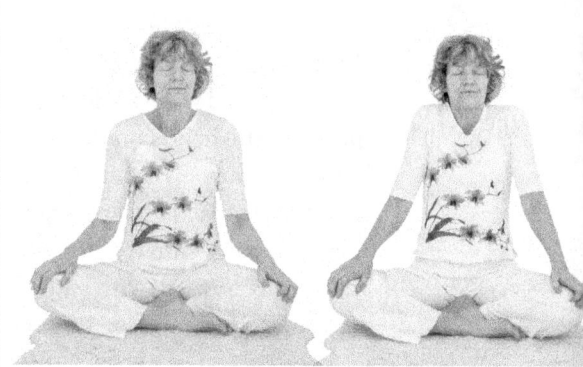

→ continue on next page

8) BABY POSE VARIATION[1].

Remain seated with the feet hip-width apart. Rest the arms on the thighs with the elbows out to the sides. Make the hands into fists, one on top of the other. Bend forward from the hips and let your forehead rest on them. Relax in this pose while breathing normally. Do this for **45 seconds**.

9) SHOULDER ROLLS.

Remain seated with the hands on the thighs. Roll the shoulders forward in large circles for **30 seconds**. Reverse the direction and roll the shoulders backward in large circles for another **30 seconds**. Breathe normally. Relax.

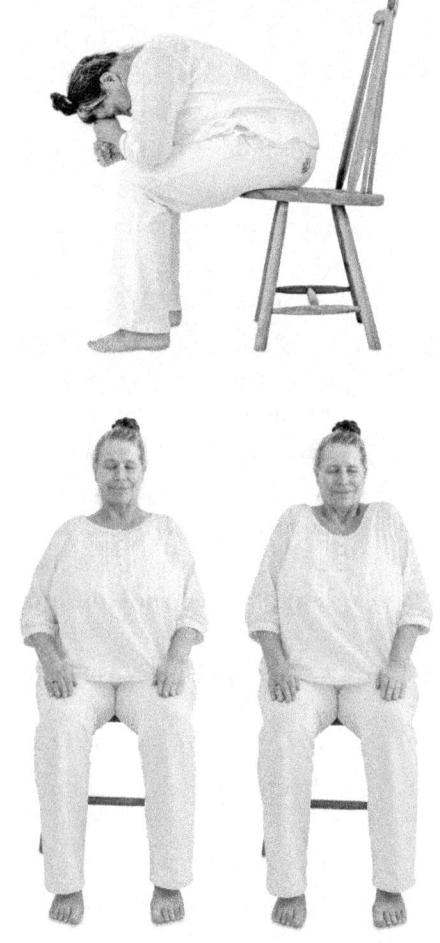

---

[1] Authors' Note: Alternative: Coachman Pose. Here the pose is more straight up, which is suitable for people with increased blood or eye pressure or for those with heart conditions. You can also use a table: you sit at a table, arms shoulder-width on the tabletop and your forehead resting on the table. Relax in this posture. In case of increased eye pressure, do not bend forward. In case of a heart condition, do not bring the head further down than the heart.

→ continue on next page

10) NECK ROLLS.

In Easy Pose, begin rolling the head in large, smooth circles in one direction, consciously relaxing the neck, throat, and shoulders. The breath is relaxed. Continue for **45 seconds**. Then reverse direction and continue for **45 seconds**.

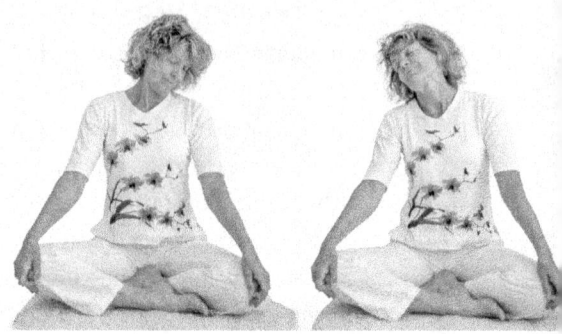

11) SITALI PRANAYAM.

Sit in Easy Pose with a straight spine and a light Neck Lock and place the hands in Gyan Mudra on the knees. Curl the tongue into a "U" shape and extend it slightly past the lips. Inhale deeply through the curled tongue, exhale through the nose. Breathe long and deep for **4 minutes**.

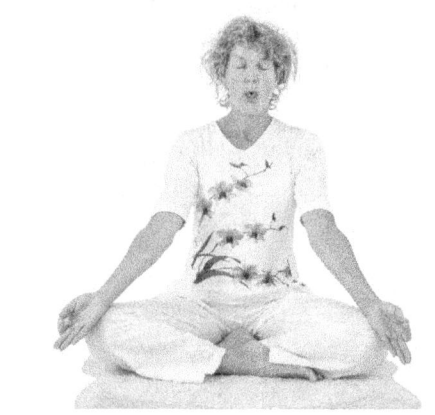

Comments: This twenty-minute series is to be done at a very slow, relaxing pace. It is a fine way to clear out the effects of a busy, stressful day.

10) HALF NECK TURN[2].

Remain seated with a straight spine and light Neck Lock. Turn the head slowly to the left as if you want to look over your shoulder as you inhale and turn back to the center as you exhale. Continue for **45 seconds**. Then reverse direction and continue for **45 seconds**.

11) SITALI PRANAYAM.

Remain seated with a straight spine and a light Neck Lock with the hands in Gyan Mudra on the knees. Curl the tongue into a "U" shape and extend it slightly past the lips. Inhale deeply through the curled tongue, exhale through the nose. Breathe long and deep for **2 minutes**.

Comments: This series is to be done at a very slow, relaxing pace. It is a fine way to clear out the effects of a busy, stressful day.

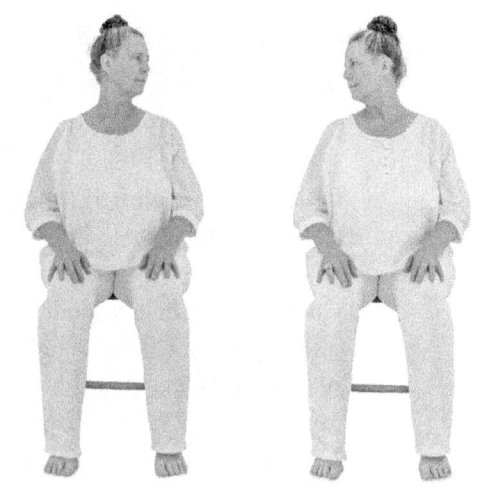

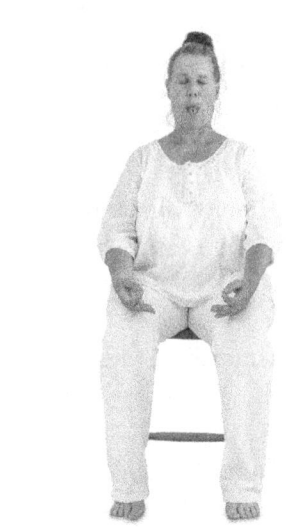

---

2   Authors' Note: When moving the head to each shoulder, maintain a light Neck Lock with the sternum lifted. Take care in the movement, so that the head does not tilt backwards. If there are any neck issues or tilting the head backward causes discomfort, limit the movement by keeping the chin on the chest or try other modifications such as drawing small circles with the nose or doing half circles from one side to the other without rolling to the back.

3.3 Meditation to Remove Fear of the Future
October 26, 1988

Sit in Easy Pose with a straight spine and a light Neck Lock.

Mudra: Place the left hand in the palm of the right hand. Grasp the left hand by curling the fingers of the right hand around the left hand and the right thumb on the left palm. Cross the left thumb over the right thumb. Hold this mudra gently at the Heart Center.

Eye Focus: Not specified.

Breath: Not specified.

Mantra: Meditate on your favorite version of the shabad **DHAN DHAN RAM DAS GUROO**.

Time: Start with **11 minutes** and slowly build to **31 minutes**.

To End: Inhale deeply, exhale. Repeat **2 more times**.

Comments: This meditation clears the fear of the future which has been created by your subconscious memories of the past. It connects you to the flow of life and to become conscious of the Self through your Heart Center. The mudra awakens a peaceful, secure feeling.

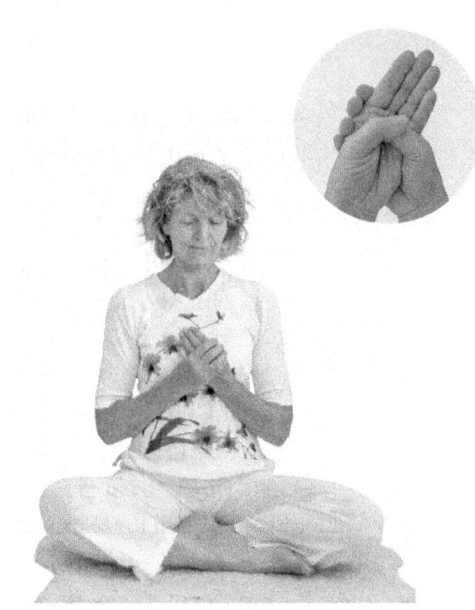

ON THE CHAIR

Sit comfortably in a chair with the weight of both feet resting evenly on the ground, with a straight spine and a light Neck Lock.

Practice as described on the side.

Time: Start with **5 ½ minutes** and gradually increase to **11 minutes**.

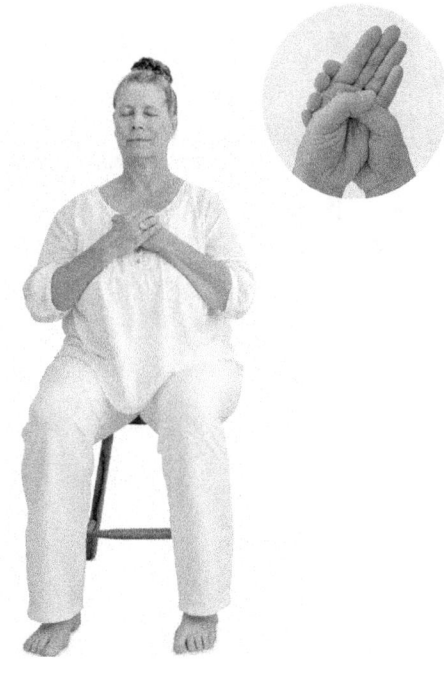

CHAPTER 4
Foundations

—

If you keep up, you shall be kept up.
— YOGI BHAJAN, JANUARY 4, 1994

In this chapter, you will begin with working on your chakras, beginning with the first chakra or the *Muladhara*. This chakra acts as the body's root and is associated with your foundation, sense of security, letting go, and acceptance. The root chakra is located near the tailbone – at the base of the spine – near the excretory organs. It relates to your connection to the earth, your ability to dig in and feel firmly grounded in your life, and thus with acceptance, self-confidence and stability, but also with the ability to let go and have healthy elimination. The first chakra has to do with being centered and also to the feeling of belonging on this Earth.

The first chakras' motto is: *I accept who I am*. The color red is associated with this chakra. The subtle perception is smell. The element is earth. Organs include the colon and rectum. Chakra imbalances in the first chakra manifest as a weakened mental and physical constitution, a sense of alienation or a feeling that you don't belong, and a proclivity for primal, animalistic responses. When out of balance, you may feel depressed, anxious, stuck, or lethargic. You may also notice a sudden increase or decrease in weight, constipation, pelvic pain, and incontinence.

In terms of childhood development, this connection to stability, security and rootedness is the first and most essential. When we are born, the upper chakra (crown chakra) is still wide open, so in some sense we are not yet of this world. The task of the parents is to support the child, to make it feel welcome on earth, and to allow it to grow and find its root in this life. As a result, the root chakra is opened. For this reason, physical contact is essential: it makes babies feel secure. This is why during the first phase of life it is critical to meet the baby's basic needs, such as food, cleaning, and touch/caring.

What affects the first chakra: exercises for your feet and legs, as well as exercises that restore contact with the earth. Scent stimulation also helps you connect and strengthen the first chakra, for example, the smell of your favorite childhood food.

The breath exercise, kriya and meditation chosen for this chapter will help you become more aware of your first chakra. The first breath practice *Long and Deep Breathing* boosts inner strength and energy by balancing the nervous system and bringing about balanced breathing. The kriya *Basic Spinal Energy Series* improves the spine's flexibility as well as increasing the energy of the chakras. It has benefits for mental clarity and memory. The meditation *Kirtan Kriya* brings total mental balance by meditating on the cycle of creation, and utilizing mudra and mantra to stimulate the psyche for greater mental focus and memory.

4.1 Long and Deep Breathing
Originally published in the Aquarian Teacher Yoga Manual

Sit straight on the ground, in a chair, or lie on the back. Initially have the left hand on the belly, right hand on the chest to feel the movement of the diaphragm.

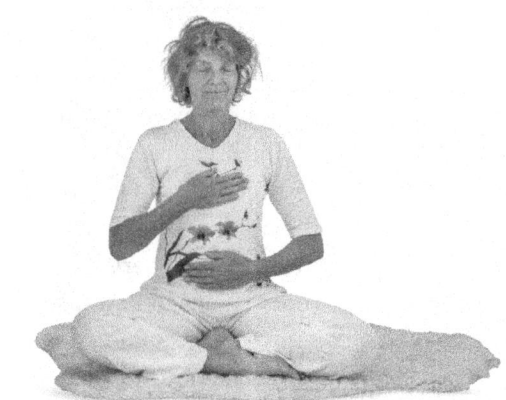

1) ABDOMINAL BREATH.
Let the breath relax to a normal pace and depth. Bring your attention to the Navel Point area. Take a slow deep breath by letting the belly relax and expand. As you exhale, gently pull the navel in and up toward the spine. For this experiment, keep the chest relaxed. Focus on breathing entirely with the lower abdomen. Place one hand on the Navel Point and one on the center of the chest. On the inhale, raise the hand on the navel toward the ceiling. On the exhale, lower it steadily. With your hand, monitor the chest to stay still and relaxed. Very soon you will notice all the muscles involved in this motion. Continue for **1-3 minutes**.

2) CHEST BREATH.
Sit straight and keep the diaphragm still. Do not let the abdomen extend. Inhale slowly using the chest muscles. The chest expands by using the intercostal muscles between the ribs. Do this slowly

→ continue on next page

ON THE CHAIR

Sit comfortably in a chair with the weight of both feet resting evenly on the ground, with a straight spine and a light Neck Lock.

Practice as described on the side.

Time: Start with **1 minute** for each of the three parts and gradually increase to **3 minutes**.

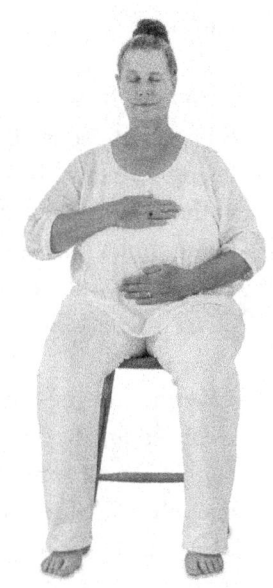

and focus on the sensation of expansion. Exhale completely but do not use the abdomen. Compare the depth and volume of this breath with the isolated abdominal breath. Continue for **1-3 minutes**.

3) CLAVICULAR BREATH.
Sit straight. Contract the navel in and keep the abdomen tight. Lift the chest without inhaling. Now inhale slowly by expanding the shoulders and the collarbone. Exhale as you keep the chest lifted. Continue for **1-3 minutes**.

Comments: The breath relaxes, cleanses, and brings you to your center. Most people do not exhale entirely, allowing consumed oxygen to remain in the lungs. Breath signatures which create shallow, erratic, upper-chest breathing are common. Therefore, it is important to breathe out properly. Of all the positive changes a person can make, learning to breathe deeply and completely is probably the most effective tool for developing higher consciousness and increasing health and vitality.

Long Deep Breathing uses the full capacity of the lungs, by utilizing the three chambers of the lungs: the abdominal or lower, the chest or middle, and the clavicular or upper. Long Deep Breathing starts by filling the abdomen, then expanding the chest, and finally lifting the upper ribs and clavicle. The exhale is the reverse: first the upper deflates, then the middle, and finally the abdomen pulls in and up, as the Navel Point pulls back toward the spine.

The Long Deep Breathing speeds up the physical and emotional healing processes, helps to break unconscious habit patterns and addictions, stimulates the production of chemicals in the brain to work against depression, reduces waste buildup in the lungs by properly opening up the air sacs, balances the parasympathetic and sympathetic nervous systems, and cleanses the blood of carbon dioxide to maintain blood homeostasis.

4.2 Basic Spinal Energy Series
Originally published in the Aquarian Teacher Yoga Manual

1) CAMEL RIDE.
Sit in Easy Pose with a straight spine and a light Neck Lock. Grasp the shins or ankles with the hands. Tilt the pelvis forward on the inhale and backward on the exhale. Only the pelvis and lower spine move. The rib cage, shoulders and head are still and remain over the hips. The motion is fluid and continuous. Repeat **108 times**. Breathe powerfully. TO END: Inhale, exhale.
Relax for **1 minute**.
Camel Ride has a "multi-stage reaction pattern" that greatly alters the proportions and strengths of alpha, theta and delta waves. It helps loosen the lower back. Making the spine more flexible has an effect on multiple levels.

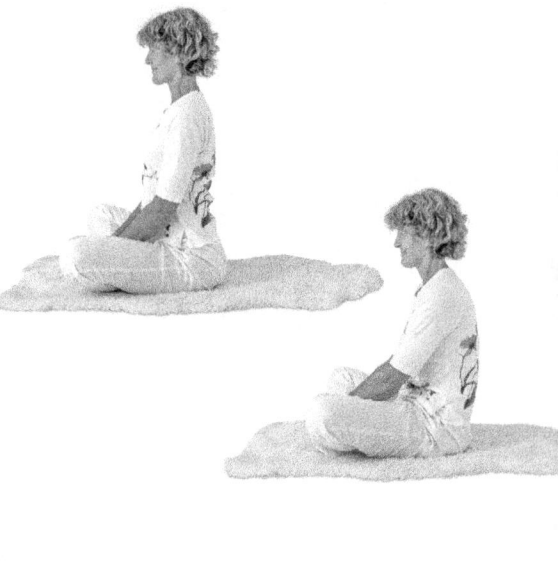

2) SPINAL FLEX IN ROCK POSE.
Sit on the heels in Rock Pose with a straight spine and a light Neck Lock. Place the hands flat on the thighs. Flex the spine forward and lift the chest on the inhale, and flex the spine backward on the exhale. The movement is at the level of the solar plexus. The rib cage, shoulders, and head are still and remain over the hips. Hands stay fixed on the thighs. Mentally vibrate **SAT** on the inhale, **NAAM** on the exhale. Repeat **108 times**.

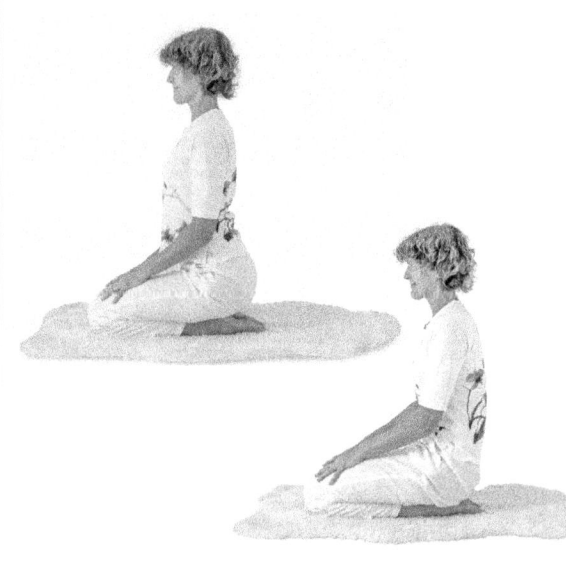

→ continue on next page

ON THE CHAIR

1) CAMEL RIDE.
Sit comfortably in a chair with feet hip-width apart, a straight spine and a light Neck Lock. Place the hands on the upper thighs at the crease of the hips. Tilt the pelvis forward on the inhale, and backward on the exhale. Only the pelvis and lower spine move. The rib cage, shoulders and head are still and remain over the hips. The motion is fluid and continuous. Repeat **26 times**. Breathe powerfully.
TO END: Inhale, exhale.
Relax for **1 minute**.
Camel Ride has a "multi-stage reaction pattern" that greatly alters the proportions and strengths of alpha, theta and delta waves. It helps loosen the lower back. Making the spine more flexible has an effect on multiple levels.

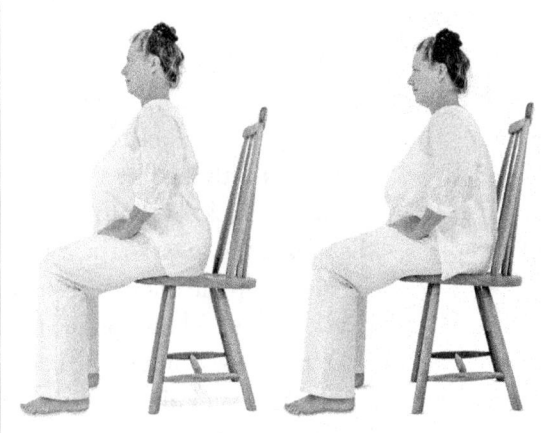

2) SPINAL FLEX.
Remain seated and place the hands on the thighs near the knees, with the shoulders relaxed. Flex the spine forward and lift the chest on the inhale, and flex the spine backward on the exhale. The movement is at the level of the solar plexus. The rib cage, shoulders, and head are still and remain over the hips. Hands stay fixed on the thighs. Mentally

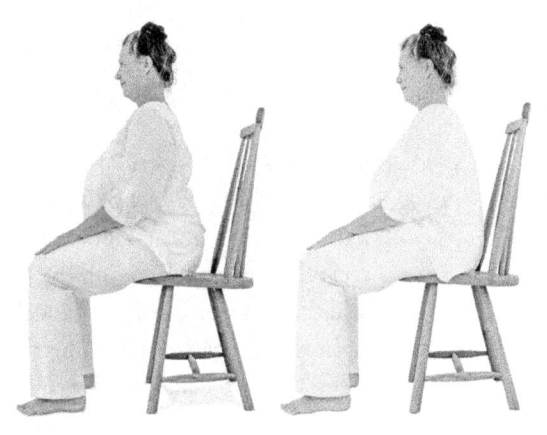

→ continue on next page

TO END: Inhale, exhale.
Relax for **2 minutes**.
Through practicing this exercise the middle part of the back and the shoulder girdle are loosened up.

3) SPINAL TWIST.

Sit in Easy Pose with a straight spine and a light neck Lock. Grasp the shoulders with the fingers in front, thumbs in back. Twist to the left on the inhale and twist to the right on the exhale. Keep the upper arms parallel to the ground, elbows pulled back to open the chest. Initiate the movement from the Navel Point, not the arms. The head moves last. Repeat **26 times**.
TO END: Inhale at the center, suspend the breath for a moment and exhale. Relax for **1 minute**.
This exercise opens the Heart Center and stimulates the upper part of the spine. It is beneficial for the nervous system, the heart and lungs; it strengthens the pectoral as well as back muscles.

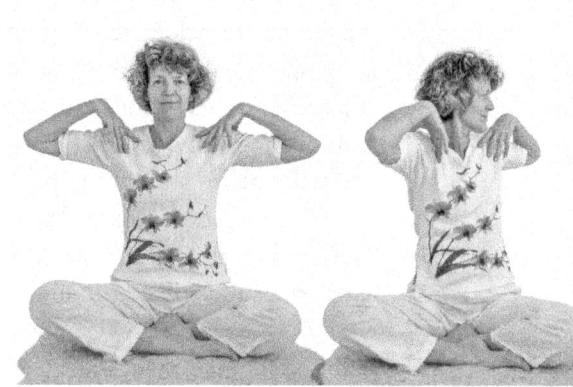

4) SEE-SAW IN BEAR GRIP.

Remain in Easy Pose. Bring the hands in front of the Heart Center with the right palm facing the body and the left facing forward; curl the right fingers in the left in Bear Grip. Keep the forearms parallel to the ground. Move the elbows in a see-saw motion, breathing deeply with the motion. Repeat **26 times**.

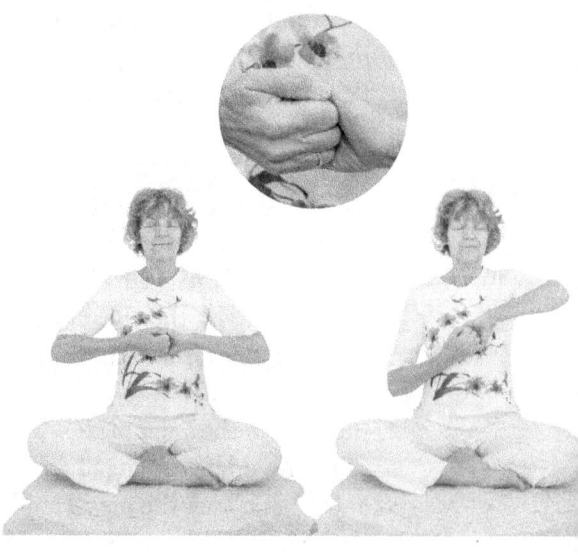

→ continue on next page

vibrate **SAT** on the inhale, **NAAM** on the exhale. Repeat **26 times**.
TO END: Inhale, exhale.
Relax for **2 minutes**.
Through practicing this exercise the middle part of the back and the shoulder girdle are loosened up.

3) SPINAL TWIST.

Remain seated and grasp the shoulders with the fingers in front, thumbs in back. Twist to the left on the inhale and twist to the right on the exhale. Keep the upper arms parallel to the ground, elbows pulled back to open the chest. Initiate the movement from the Navel Point, not the arms. The head moves last. If there is a back condition, move gently with care. Repeat **6 times**.
TO END: Inhale at the center, suspend the breath for a moment and exhale. Relax for **1 minute**.
This exercise opens the Heart Center and stimulates the upper part of the spine. It is beneficial for the nervous system, the heart and lungs; it strengthens the pectoral as well as back muscles.

4) SEE-SAW IN BEAR GRIP.

Remain seated. Bring the hands in front of the Heart Center with the right palm facing the body and the left facing forward; curl the right fingers in the left in Bear Grip. Keep the forearms parallel to the ground. Move the elbows in a

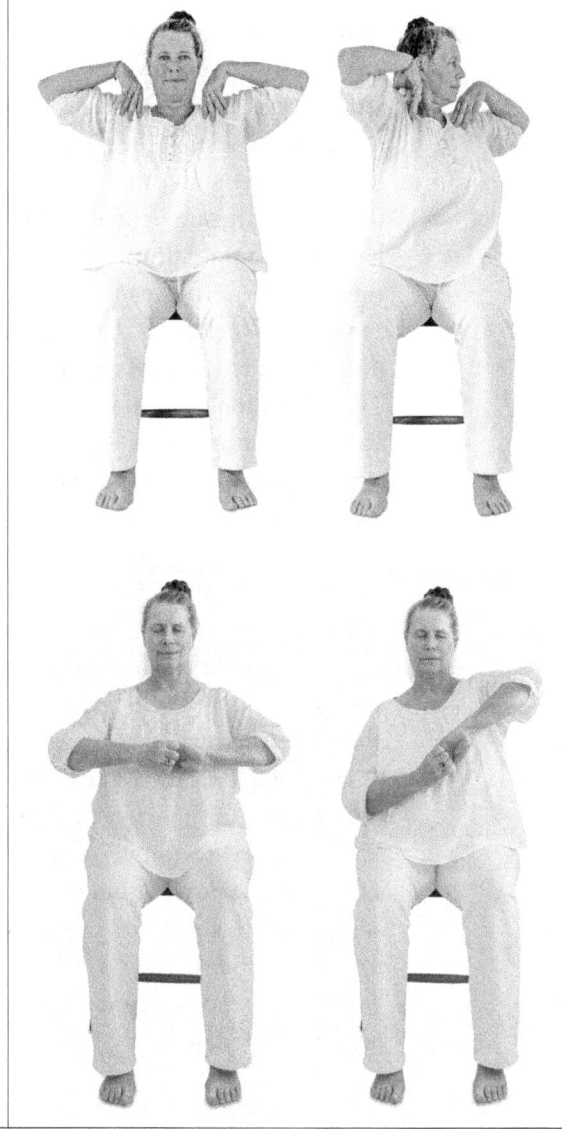

→ continue on next page

TO END: Inhale, exhale, pull the fingers. Relax **30 seconds**.
The exercise is beneficial for the Heart Center and will loosen up the back at the level of the thoracic vertebra.

5) SPINAL FLEX.
Remain in Easy Pose. Grasp the knees firmly. Keeping the elbows straight, flex the upper spine forward and lift the chest on the inhale, and flex the upper spine backward on the exhale. The movement is at the level of the upper thoracic spine in the heart area. The head is still and remains in Neck Lock. Continue at a moderate pace for **108 repetitions**.
TO END: Inhale, exhale.
Relax for **1 minute**.
It is beneficial for the upper part of the back and for the shoulders.

6) SHOULDER SHRUGS.
Remain in Easy Pose with a straight spine and a light Neck Lock. Rest the hands on the knees. Raise both shoulders up towards the ears on the inhale, drop the shoulders down on the exhale. Continue for **2 minutes**. Move and breathe powerfully.
TO END: Inhale and hold **15 seconds** with shoulders raised up, exhale, and relax.
The exercise relaxes the shoulders, neck and upper back.

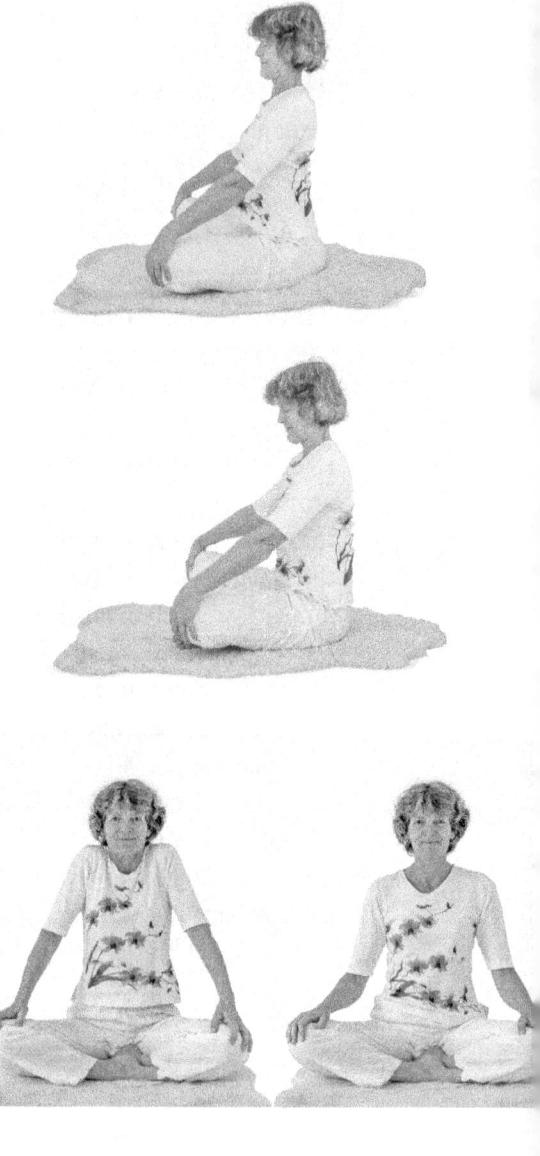

→ continue on next page

see-saw motion, breathing deeply with the motion. Repeat **6 times**.
TO END: Inhale, exhale, pull the fingers. Relax **30 seconds**.
The exercise is beneficial for the Heart Center and will loosen up the back at the level of the thoracic vertebra.

5) SPINAL FLEX.

Remain seated with the hands on the thighs, keep the arms straight and the shoulders relaxed. Flex the upper spine forward, lifting the chest on the inhale and flexing the upper spine backward on the exhale. The movement is at the level of the upper thoracic spine in the heart area. The head is still and remains in Neck Lock. Continue at a moderate pace for **26 times**.
TO END: Inhale, exhale.
Relax for **1 minute**.
It is beneficial for the upper part of the back and for the shoulders.

6) SHOULDER SHRUGS.

Remain seated with the hands on the thighs, keep the arms straight. Raise both shoulders up towards the ears on the inhale, lower the shoulders on the exhale. If you have a shoulder injury, move with care. Continue for **1 minute**.
TO END: Inhale and hold **15 seconds** with shoulders raised up, exhale, and relax.
The exercise relaxes the shoulders, neck and upper back.

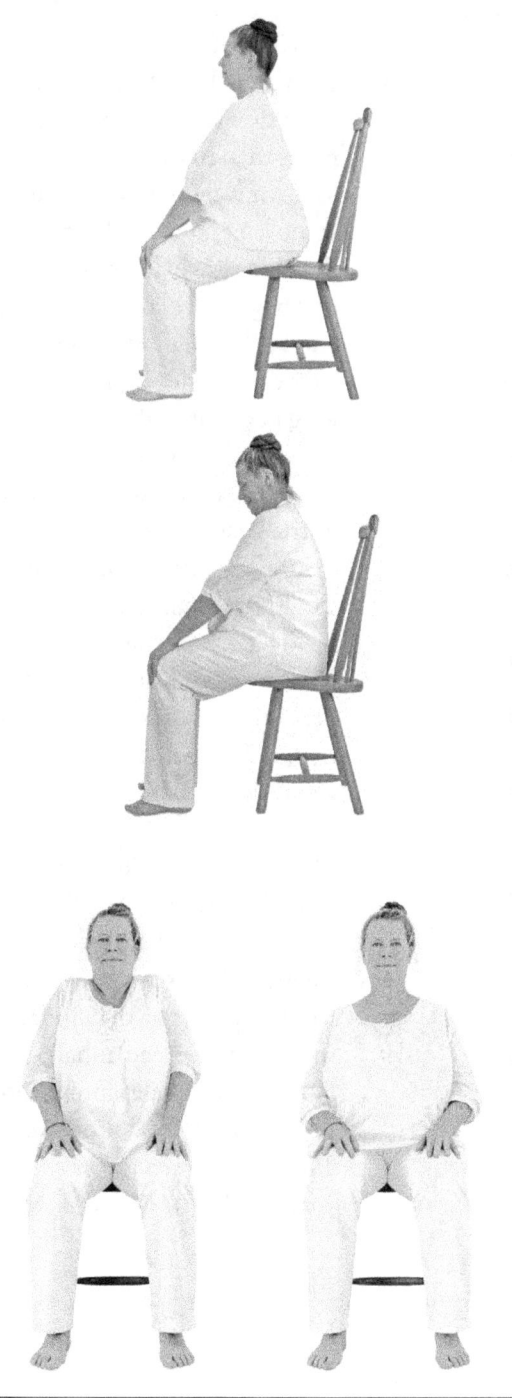

→ continue on next page

7) NECK ROLLS.

Remain in Easy Pose. Rotate the neck slowly around **5 times** to the right, then to the left **5 times** in the following manner: Inhale, lengthen the spine a bit more, and exhale, letting the chin slowly lower forward. Inhale and begin to roll the head to the side and back, exhale and continue rolling to the other side and front, keeping a long neck throughout. The shoulders remain relaxed and stable, and the neck should be allowed to gently stretch as the head circles around. Continue in a slow and smooth motion.
TO END: Inhale and float the head back up to neutral.
This exercise is beneficial for the neck and throat area; it releases tension in the neck and stimulates circulation toward the head.

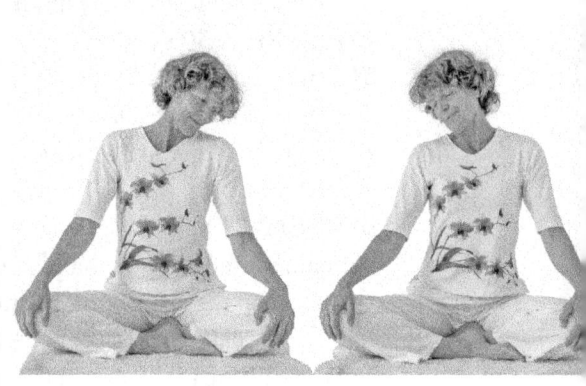

8) BEAR GRIP VARIATION.

Remain in Easy Pose. Place the hands into a Bear Grip at the throat level. Inhale, apply Root Lock, exhale, apply Root Lock. Raise the mudra above the top of the head, inhale, apply Root Lock, exhale, apply Root Lock. Repeat the cycle **2 more times**.
Through this exercise the energy in your body starts to flow again.

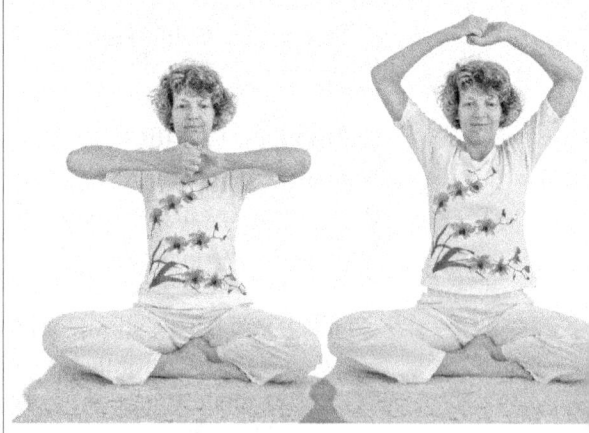

→ continue on next page

7) HALF NECK ROLL[1].

Remain seated. Stretch the spine, slightly lift the back of the head, making the neck long. On the inhale, move your head slowly to the left, as if trying to look over your shoulder; while exhaling come back to the center. Continue for **3 times**. Then change sides and continue for **3 times**.
TO END: Inhale and float the head back up to neutral.
This exercise is beneficial for the neck and throat area; it releases tension in the neck and stimulates circulation toward the head.

8) BEAR GRIP VARIATION.

Remain seated. Place the hands into a Bear Grip at the throat level. Inhale, apply Root Lock, exhale, apply Root Lock. Raise the mudra above the top of the head, inhale, apply Root Lock, exhale, apply Root Lock. Repeat the cycle **1 more time**.
Through this exercise the energy in your body starts to flow again.

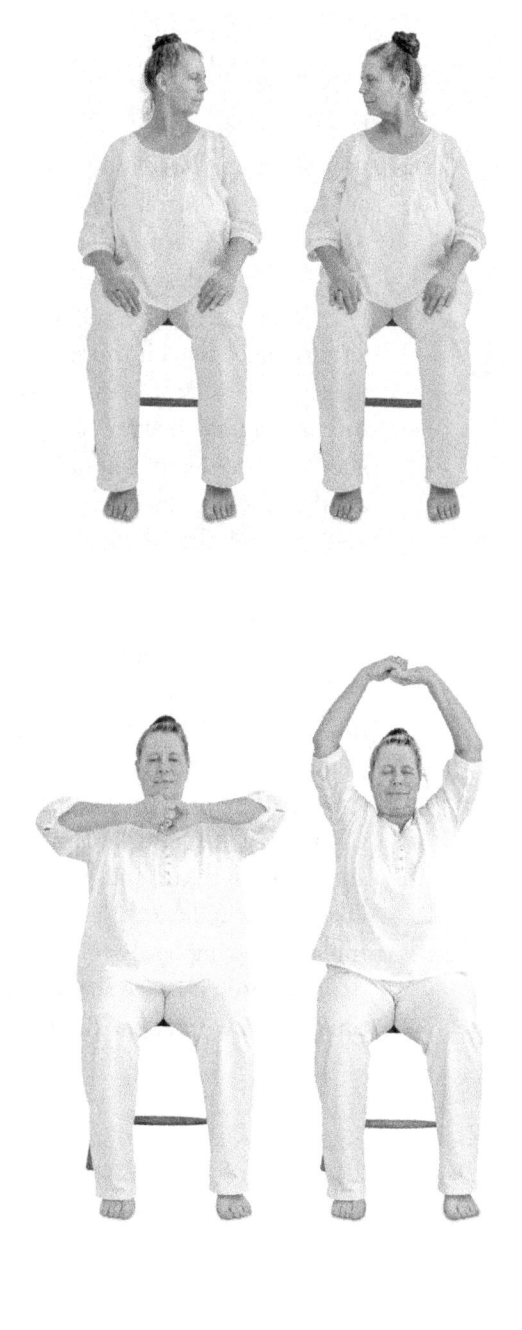

---

1 Authors' Note: When moving the head to each shoulder, maintain a light Neck Lock with the sternum lifted. Take care in the movement, so that the head does not tilt backwards. If there are any neck issues or tilting the head backward causes discomfort, limit the movement by keeping the chin on the chest or try other modifications such as drawing small circles with the nose or doing half circles from one side to the other without rolling to the back.

→ continue on next page

9) SAT KRIYA.
Sit on the heels in Rock Pose with a straight spine and a light Neck Lock. Interlace the fingers with the Jupiter (index) fingers pointing up and the thumbs crossed. For working with masculine, projective energy, place the right thumb over the left. For working feminine, reflective energy, place the left thumb over the right. Reach the arms overhead, roll the armpits forward, keeping the shoulders down; the shoulder blades are drawn down and wide. Chant **SAT** and pull the Navel Point in and up. Chant **NAAM** as you release it. Continue rhythmically for **3 minutes**. TO END: Inhale, apply Root Lock and squeeze the muscles tightly from the buttocks all the way up the spine. Mentally allow the energy to flow through the top of the skull. Exhale completely, suspend the breath out and apply all three locks (Root Lock, Diaphragm Lock and Neck Lock). Inhale and completely relax. Ideally the relaxation is twice the length of time that you practiced Sat Kriya.

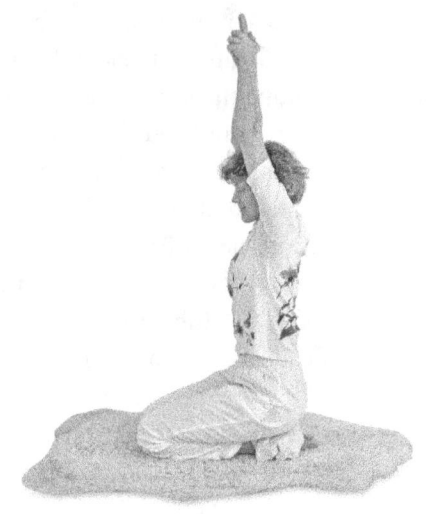

→ continue on next page

9) SAT KRIYA[2].

Remain seated with the feet hip-width apart and a light Neck Lock. Interlace the fingers with the Jupiter (index) fingers pointing up and the thumbs crossed. For working with masculine, projective energy, place the right thumb over the left. For working feminine, reflective energy, place the left thumb over the right. Stretch the arms straight up past the ears while keeping the palms together[3]. Chant **SAT** and pull the Navel Point in and up. Chant **NAAM** as you release it. Continue rhythmically for **1 minute**. TO END: Inhale, apply Root Lock and squeeze the muscles tightly from the buttocks all the way up the spine. Suspend the breath briefly as you concentrate on the area just above the top of the head. Mentally allow the energy to flow through the top of the skull. Exhale completely. Inhale, exhale, suspend the breath for **5-20 seconds** and apply all three locks, the Great Lock (Root Lock, Diaphragm Lock and Neck Lock[4]). Inhale and completely relax for **2 minutes**.

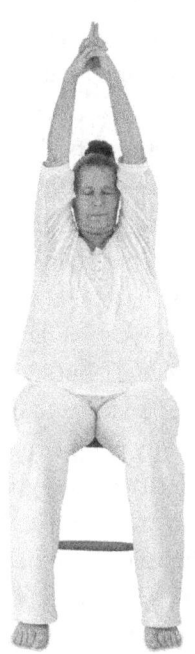

---

2 Authors' Note: While performing the exercise, all organs will receive a soft, rhythmic massage. The heart will be strengthened. People who are unbalanced or have mental health issues might benefit from Sat Kriya. Do not forget to relax after this exercise.

3 Authors' Note: If this is not possible, leave your hands in your lap and practice the exercise in your mind.

4 Please check initial pages, page 18, to review full instructions on each one of the Body Locks.

→ continue on next page

10) RELAXATION.
Lie down on the back in Corpse Pose and relax for **15 minutes**.

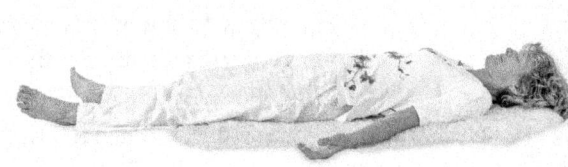

Comments: Age is measured by the flexibility of the spine: to stay young, stay flexible. This kriya works systematically from the base of the spine to the top. All 26 vertebrae receive stimulation and all the chakras receive a burst of energy. This makes it a good kriya to do before meditation. Many people report greater mental clarity after regular practice of this kriya. A contributing factor is the increased circulation of the spinal fluid, which is crucially linked to having a good memory. In a beginner's class, each exercise that lists 108 repetitions can be done **26 times**. The rest periods are then extended from **1** to **2 minutes**.

10) RELAXATION.

Sit comfortably in the back of the chair, the lower back well supported. Keep your feet on the ground and connect with the earth. Place your hands on the upper legs, palms up. Relax for **15 minutes**.

Comments: Age is measured by the flexibility of the spine: to stay young, stay flexible. This kriya works systematically from the base of the spine to the top. All 26 vertebrae receive stimulation and all the chakras receive a burst of energy. This makes it a good kriya to do before meditation. Many people report greater mental clarity after regular practice of this kriya. A contributing factor is the increased circulation of the spinal fluid, which is crucially linked to having a good memory.

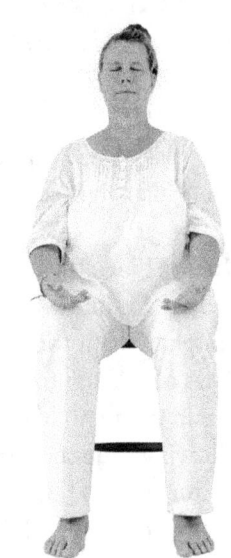

4.3 Kirtan Kriya Meditation
Originally published in the Aquarian Teacher Yoga Manual

Sit in Easy Pose with a straight spine and a light Neck Lock.

Mudra: Place the hands on the knees in Gyan Mudra with the elbows straight. Chant the mantra **SAA TAA NAA MAA** and touch the tip of the thumb to the tip of each finger in the following sequence: thumb tip to the Jupiter (index) finger on **SAA**, thumb tip to Saturn (middle) finger on **TAA**, thumb tip to Sun (ring) finger on **NAA** and thumb tip to Mercury (little) finger on **MAA**. Each repetition of the entire mantra takes **3 to 4 seconds**.

Eye Focus: Third Eye Point.

Breath: Not specified.

Mantra: SAA TAA NAA MAA. Chant aloud for **5 minutes**. Then whisper for **5 minutes**. Then go deeply into silence, mentally vibrating the sound for **10 minutes**. Then whisper for **5 minutes**. Then chant aloud for **5 minutes**.

Visualization: Meditate on the primal sounds in the "L" form. Guide the constant inflow of cosmic energy into the top of the head, the Crown Chakra. As the energy enters the head,

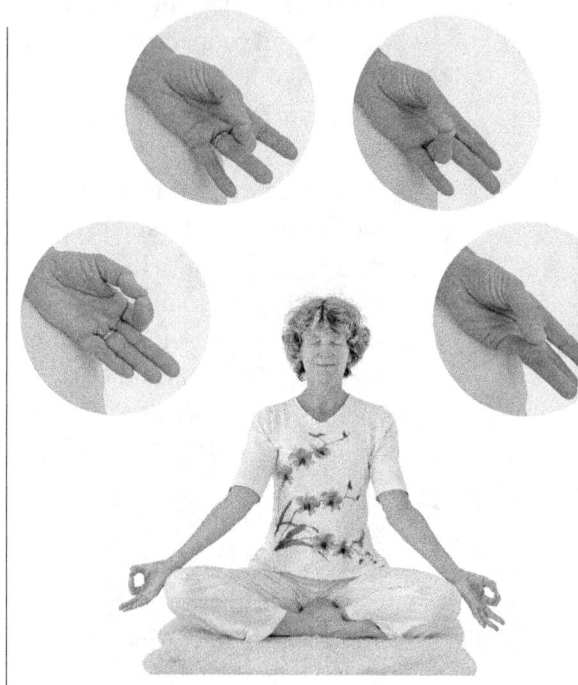

→ continue on next page

ON THE CHAIR

Sit comfortably in a chair with the weight of both feet resting evenly on the ground, with a straight spine and a light Neck Lock.

Practice as described on the side, adapting the time to the following pattern.

Time: Start the kriya with a normal voice and continue for **1 minute**; then whisper for **1 minute**; then mentally vibrate for **2 minutes**. Start whispering again for **1 minute**, then out loud again for **1 minute**.

Comments: The duration of the mediation may vary, as long as the proportions of aloud, whisper, silent, whisper, aloud are maintained. For example, 2 minutes aloud, 2 minutes whisper, 4 minutes silent, 2 minutes whisper and 2 minutes aloud.

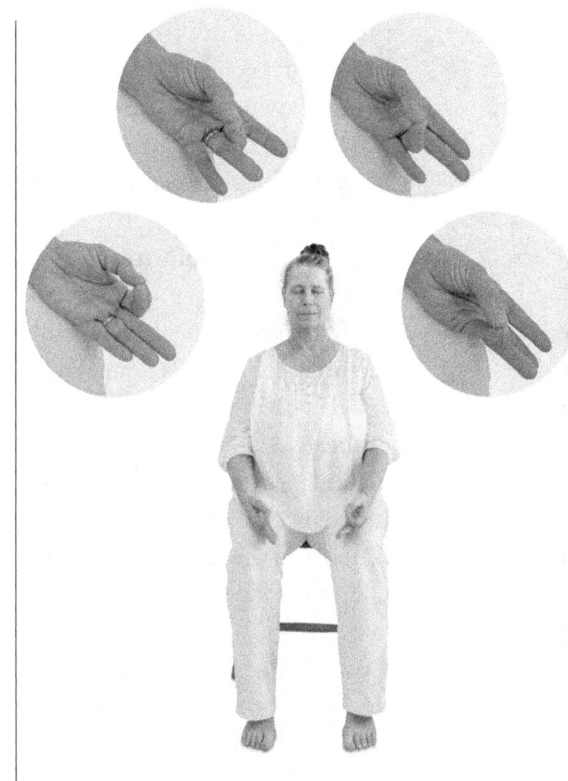

guide the sounds **SAA, TAA, NAA,** or **MAA**. As you chant **SAA** for example, the "S" starts above your head and the "A" moves down to the center of the head and out through the Third Eye Point, projected to Infinity. This energy flow follows the pathway called the Golden Cord—the connection between the pineal and pituitary gland.

Total Time: 30 minutes.

To End: Inhale deeply, suspend the breath as long as comfortable, exhale completely. Meditate in absolute stillness and silence or mentally say a prayer for **1 minute**. Elongate the spine, stretch the arms up, spread the fingers wide and take several deep breaths. Relax.

Comments: This kriya uses the five primal sounds in the original *bij* form of the word "Sat Naam." Where **SAA** stands for "Infinity, cosmos, beginning," **TAA** for "life, existence," **NAA** for "death, change, transformation" and **MAA** for "Rebirth." This is the cycle of creation. From the Infinite comes life and individual existence. From life comes death or change. From death comes the rebirth of consciousness. From rebirth comes the joy of the Infinite through which compassion leads back to life.

Practicing this meditation brings a total mental balance to the individual psyche. Do this as often as necessary to stay alert. Practicing this meditation is both a science and an art. It is an art in the way it both molds consciousness and produces a refinement of sensation and insight. It is a science in the tested certainty of the results it brings about[5].

The timing can be decreased or increased as long as you maintain the ratio of spoken, whispered, and silent chanting—always ending with 1 minute of complete stillness and silence. Through this constant practice, the mind awakens to the infinite capacity of the soul for sacrifice, service, and creation.

---

5 Kirtan Kriya is the most researched meditation in Kundalini Yoga, with peer-reviewed studies in caregivers and in Alzheimer patients. Please check Alzheimer's Research & Prevention Foundation website at https://alzheimersprevention.org/research/kirtan-kriya-yoga-exercise/ and a research piece on our KRI blog https://kundaliniresearchinstitute.org/en/research-on-kirtan-kriya-hot-off-the-press/ [Editor's Note]

CHAPTER 5
Enjoyment

—

Happiness is your birthright. Don't let it go!

— YOGI BHAJAN, JANUARY 4, 1992

This chapter will focus on your second chakra, the *Svadhisthana*, which is located near the reproductive organs and the sacrum. The sacral chakra's primary function is feeling, overall enjoyment of life, and pleasure. When functioning properly, you can have harmonious, nurturing, and fulfilling relationships with yourself and others. As it is associated with the element of water, it represents flow, flexibility, and freedom of expression. The second chakra is associated with sexual functions that are positive, balanced, and relaxed, as well as with healthy, responsible relationships. Sensuality, creativity, reproduction, patience, enjoyment, and passion are all associated with this chakra. The second chakra in its fullness is authentic intimacy. This chakra's mottos are: *To feel, to desire, to create,* as well as the *Desire to merge.* Orange is the color associated with this chakra. The element is water. The subtle perception is taste. The organs associated with it are the reproductive organs, kidneys, and bladder. This chakra's imbalances can manifest as low self-esteem, lack of boundaries, lack of passion and feeling, rigid and withdrawn emotions, a sense of guilt, and in the physical sphere with kidney and bladder problems. Life lacks emotion and is pale in comparison to the vivid creative energy of the balanced second chakra.

In terms of childhood development, as soon as a child discovers they can influence their surroundings, the second chakra begins to open up. The child recognizes that they can be creative and either make or break something, such as building a block tower and then knocking it down. Children can feel physically excited with new experiences and with the ability to create.

What affects this chakra: exercises that strengthen the pelvis, kriyas that work on the kidneys and bladder, kriyas related to stress, and those that balance the reproductive system or sexual energy and bring rejuvenation and vitality. Also kriyas and meditations for balancing emotions are helpful for this chakra, as well as life creative expression in art, and other activities that increase flow all develop the energy in this chakra.

The breath, kriya, and meditation selected for this chapter help you connect to your second chakra, relate to the life themes associated with it, and become aware of its balanced or unbalanced functions. The breath practice *Sitali Kriya: Cooling and Calming Breath* creates awareness and makes you calmer. It is known as a cooling breath, with rejuvenating and detoxifying functions that also tonifies the kidneys, adrenals and digestive system. The *Kriya for Adrenals and Kidneys* affects creativity, your reproductive organs, and helps to channel stress. It allows for greater flow of the water element in your body. Therefore, drinking plenty of water supports this process. The *Antar Naad Mudra* meditation allows you to recognize the less desirable aspects of life. Additionally, this meditation increases creativity and enables your emotions to flow, which are hallmark aspects of the balanced second chakra.

5.1 Sitali Kriya: Cooling and Calming Breath
July 30, 1975

Sit in Easy Pose with a straight spine and a light Neck Lock.

Mudra: Place your hands in Gyan Mudra on your knees or relaxed in your lap.

Eye Focus: Not specified.

Breath: Curl the tongue into a "U" shape and extend it slightly past the lips. Inhale deeply through the curled tongue, exhale through the nose. Breathe long and deep.

Time: Minimum of **3 minutes**.

Comments: This is an excellent kriya to do before chanting the *Siri Gaitri* mantra (Raa Maa Daa Saa, Saa Say So Hung). It is also good to do it 26 times in the morning and 26 times in the evening. This kriya gives you power, strength, and vitality. Whenever you get a fever, sickness, discomfort, do this kriya. It is very cooling and it is a cure from within. At first, the tongue will taste bitter, but with practice the taste of the tongue will become sweet. It works on the kidneys, the adrenals, and the urinary system. This breath cleanses the spleen, liver, and digestive system. It also works on testosterone and the pituitary. Great powers of rejuvenation and detoxification are attributed to this breath when practiced regularly. It soothes and cools the spine in the area of the fourth, fifth, and sixth vertebrae which regulates sexual and digestive energy.

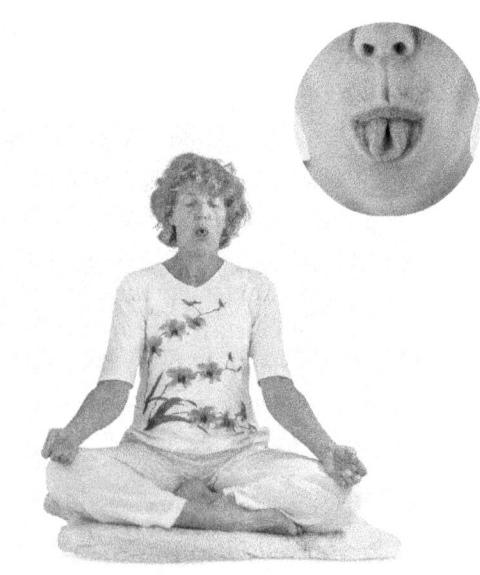

ON THE CHAIR

Sit comfortably in a chair with the weight of both feet resting evenly on the ground, with a straight spine and a light Neck Lock.

Practice as described on the side.

Time: Start with **1 minute** and gradually increase to **3 minutes**.

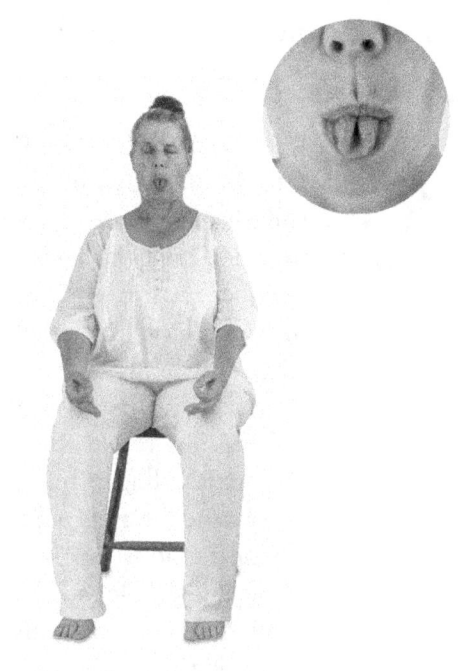

5.2 Kriya for Adrenals & Kidneys
Originally published in the Aquarian Teacher Yoga Manual

There is very little rest between the exercises.

1) LOTUS MUDRA VARIATION.
Sit in Easy Pose with a straight spine and a light Neck Lock. Rub the palms together. Bring the base of the palms together, the tips of the thumbs and Mercury (little) fingers touching, with space between the palms, and the remaining fingers stretched open in Lotus Mudra. No other part of the hands or fingers touch. Inhale as you extend the arms out to the sides, parallel to the ground, with palms facing out. Exhale as you bring the hands together into Lotus Mudra. Move rhythmically for **1-3 minutes**.
TO END: Inhale with hands in Lotus Mudra, exhale.

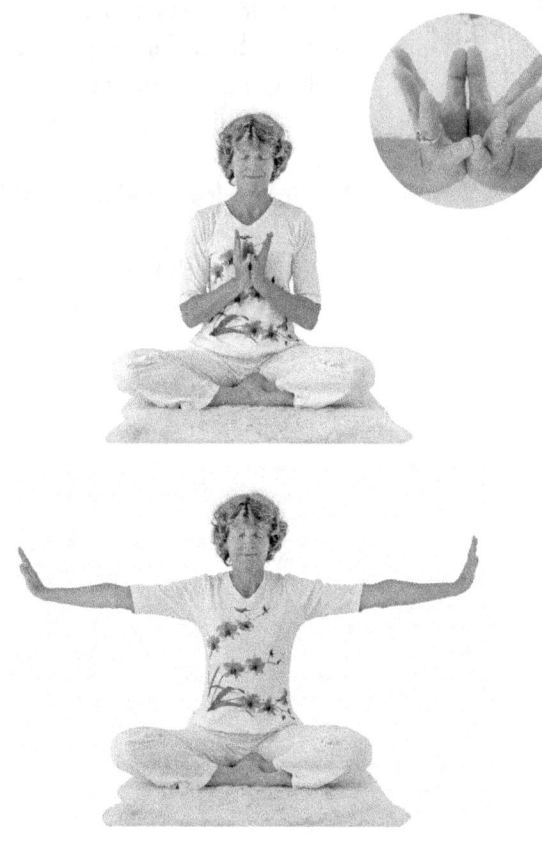

→ continue on next page

ON THE CHAIR

There is little rest between the exercises.

1) LOTUS MUDRA.
Sit in a chair, feet hip-width apart and even weight on both feet with a straight spine and a light Neck Lock. Bring the base of the palms together, thumbs and Mercury (little) fingers touching and the remaining fingers stretched open in Lotus Mudra. No other part of the hands or fingers touch. Inhale and extend the arms out to the sides, parallel to the ground, with palms facing out. Exhale and bring the hands together into Lotus Mudra. Move rhythmically for **1 minute**.
TO END: Inhale with hands in Lotus Mudra, exhale.

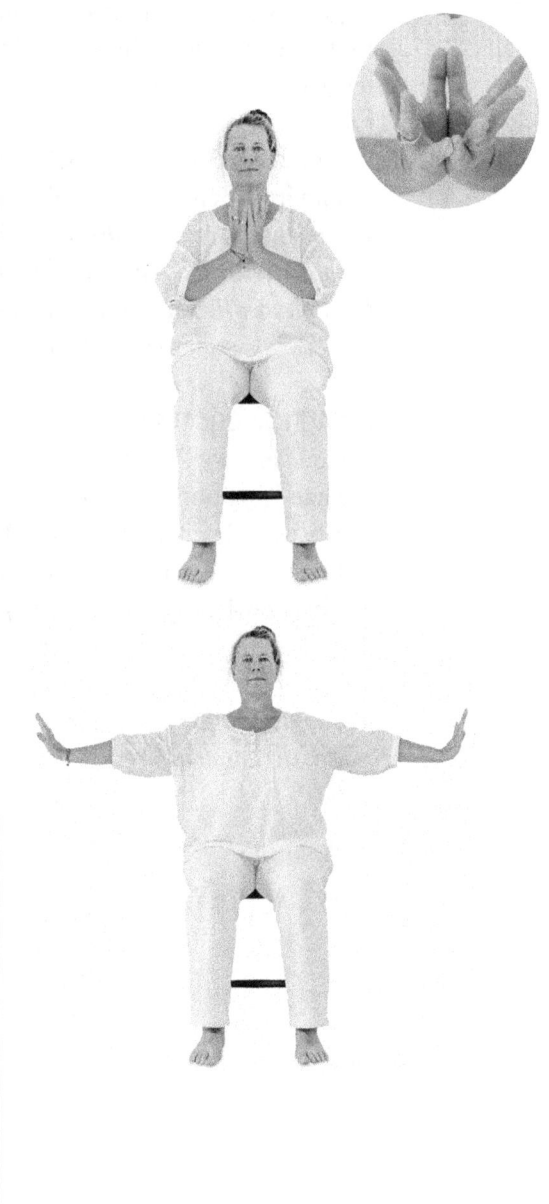

→ continue on next page

2) BREATH OF FIRE FOR THE ADRENALS.

Remain in Easy Pose. Interlock the Mercury (little) fingers in front of the Heart Center, curling the other fingers into pads, thumbs pointing up. Lower the hands to the solar plexus level and pull on the Mercury (little) fingers. Feel a pull across the back. Continue for **1-3 minutes** with Breath of Fire from below the Navel Point.
It's common for the hands to drift up. Make sure the hands are in front of the solar plexus. This generates heat and works on one side of the adrenals.

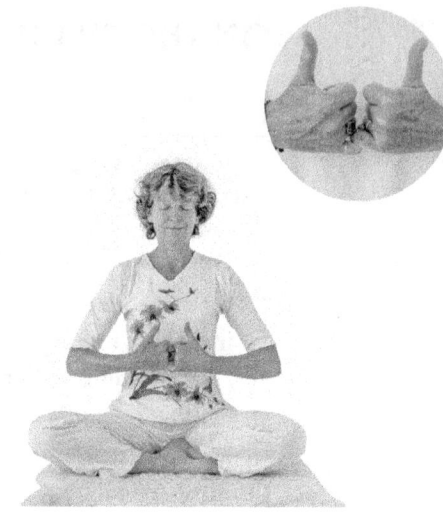

3) CANNON BREATH FOR THE ADRENALS.

Remain in Easy Pose and maintain the hand position. Continue for **1-3 minutes** with Cannon Breath. (Breath of Fire through a firm "O" mouth; don't allow the cheeks to move.)
TO END: Inhale and concentrate on the spine, exhale.
This exercise affects the other side of the adrenals.

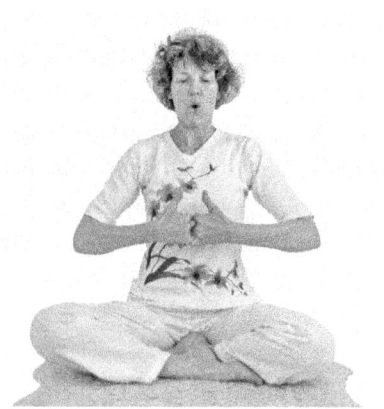

→ continue on next page

2) BREATH OF FIRE FOR THE ADRENALS.
Remain seated with the feet hip-width apart and a straight spine. Interlock the Mercury (little) fingers in front of the Heart Center, curling the other fingers into the pads, thumbs pointing up. Lower the hands to the solar plexus level and pull on the Mercury (little) fingers. Feel the pull across the back. Continue for **1 minute** with Breath of Fire from below the Navel Point.
It's common for the hands to drift up. Make sure the hands are in front of the solar plexus. This generates warmth and affects one side of the adrenal glands.

3) CANNON BREATH FOR THE ADRENALS.
Remain seated and maintain the hand position. Continue for **1 minute** with Cannon Breath. (Breath of Fire through a firm "O" mouth; don't allow the cheeks to move.)
TO END: Inhale and concentrate on the spine, exhale.
This exercise affects the other side of the adrenal glands.

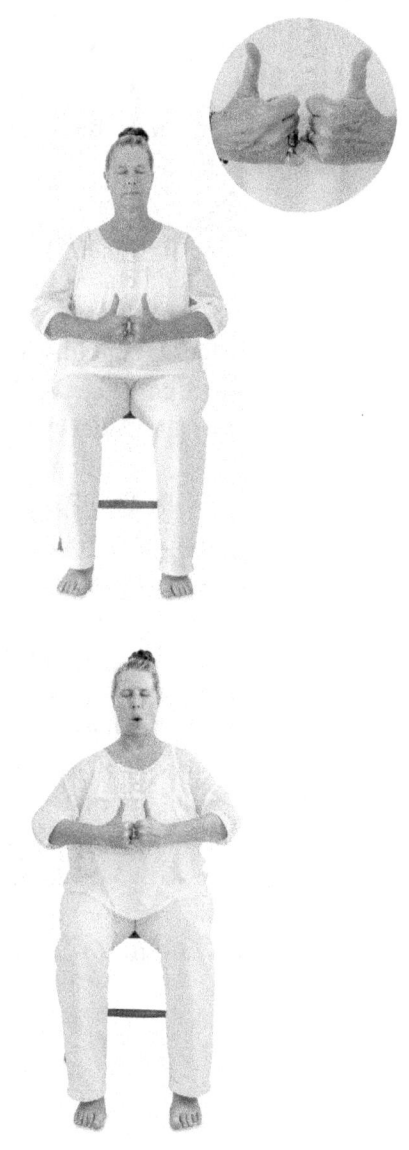

→ continue on next page

4) RIGHT ARM FORWARD CHANTING.
Remain in Easy Pose. Place the left hand on the back at the bottom rib, with the palm facing out. Extend the right arm forward, parallel to the ground. Flex the wrist and raise the hand up to a 60-degree angle. Keeping the spine straight, stretch from the shoulder. With eyes wide open, chant **HAR**, powerfully from the navel. Continue for **1-3 minutes**.

5) BODY DROPS.
Sit in Lotus Pose – if not possible, in half Lotus Pose – with a straight spine and a light Neck Lock. Place the hands on the ground next to the hips. Keeping the back straight, feet on the ground, lift the body up on the inhale and then drop it down on the exhale. Continue for **1-3 minutes**. *Spinal alignment is very important here. Keep Neck Lock applied and spine erect. Keep the back molars together to protect the tongue.*

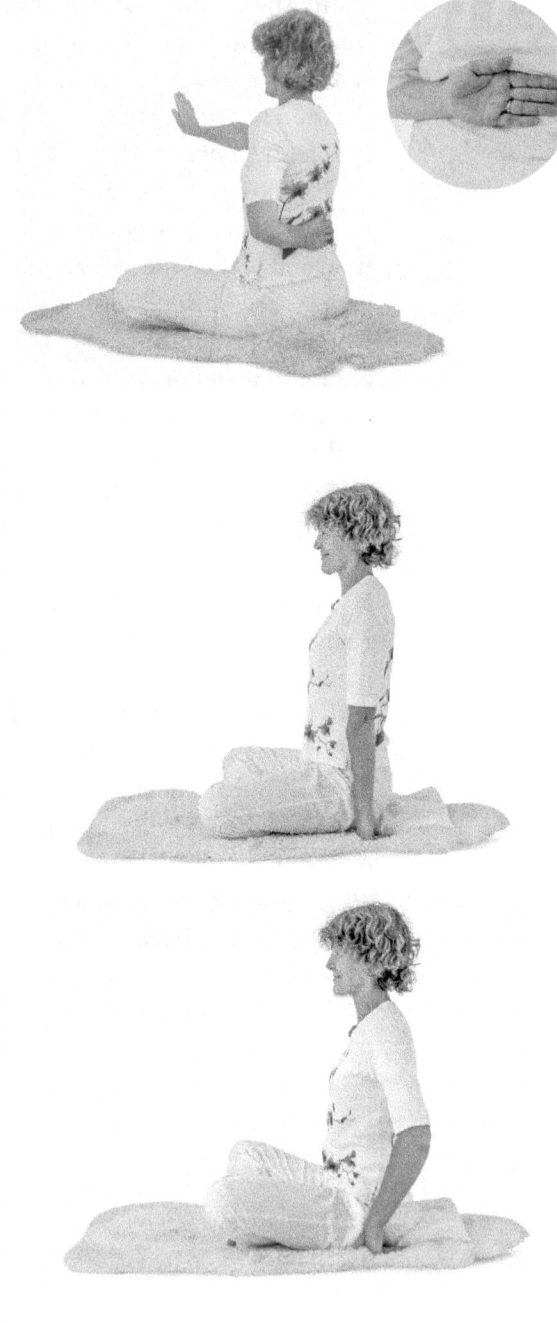

→ continue on next page

4) RIGHT ARM FORWARD CHANTING.

Remain seated with a straight spine. Place your left hand on your back at the level of the lowest rib, with the palm facing out. Extend the right arm straight forward, parallel to the ground. Flex the wrist and raise the hand up to a 60-degree angle. Keep the spine straight and stretch from the shoulder. With the eyes wide open, chant **HAR** powerfully from the navel. Continue for **1 minute**.

5) BODY DROPS.

Remain seated with a straight spine and the feet next to each other. Place the hands on the seat of the chair by your sides, or place the forearms on the armrests. Inhale, push the knees together and simultaneously squeeze the pelvic floor muscles, while making a movement as if you're getting up from the chair. It is alright to slightly come off the chair, but it is not mandatory. Exhale and relax. Continue for **1 minute**.
Spinal alignment is very important here. Keep Neck Lock applied and spine erect. Keep the back molars together to protect the tongue.

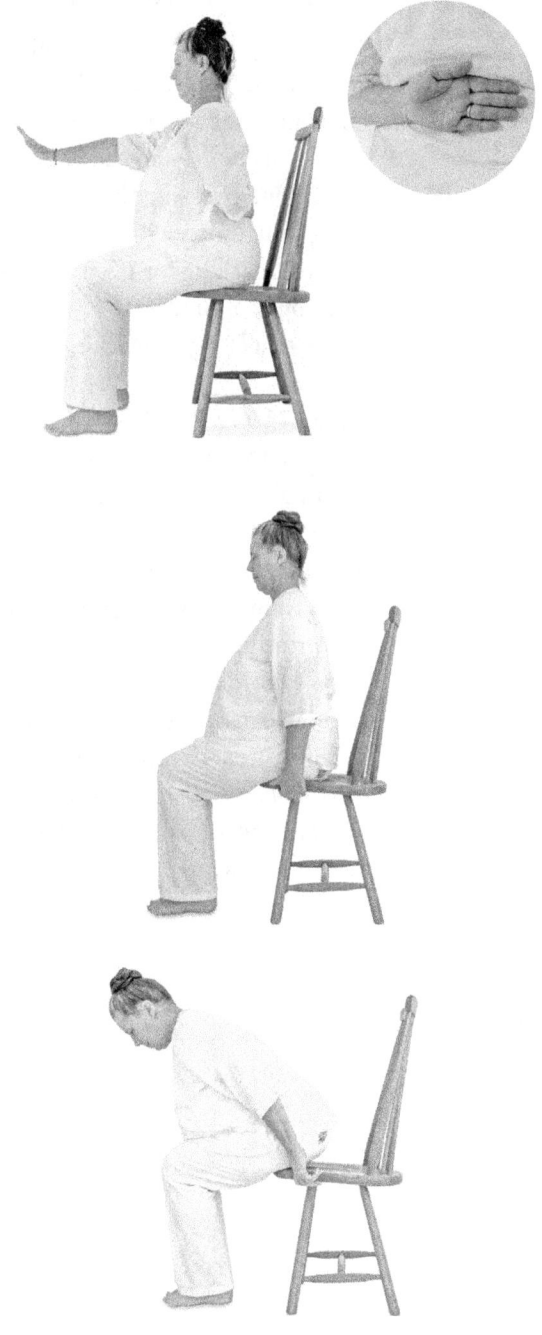

→ continue on next page

6) RIGHT HAND ON THE LEFT WRIST.
Sit in Easy Pose with a straight spine and a light Neck Lock. Place the hands in front of the solar plexus, left hand facing the body, and the base of the right hand pressing the left wrist. Eyes look down with powerful Long Deep Breathing for **1-3 minutes**.
The power of the breath is the depth to which you will cleanse.

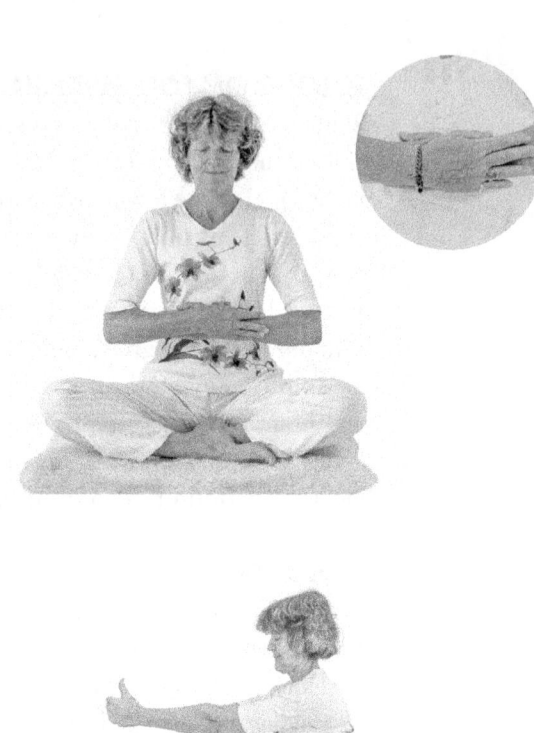

7) SEATED PARALLEL STRETCH.
Sit with the legs stretched forward, a straight spine, and a light Neck Lock. Stretch the arms forward parallel to the ground, hands in fists, thumbs pointing up. Maintain the arms parallel to the ground and inhale as you stretch forward, exhale as you lean backward. Continue for **1-3 minutes**. Breathe powerfully.
It is common to see the arms drop on the forward motion and lift on the backward motion.

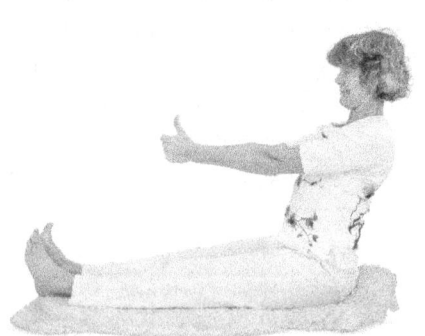

→ continue on next page

6) RIGHT HAND ON THE LEFT WRIST.
Remain seated with a straight spine and light Neck Lock. Place the hands in front of the solar plexus, left palm facing the body, and the base of the right hand pressing the left wrist. Eyes look down with powerful Long Deep Breathing for **1 minute**.
The power of the breath is the depth to which you will cleanse.

7) SEATED PARALLEL STRETCH[1].
Sit slightly forward on the seat of the chair with a straight spine. Place the right foot flat on the ground and stretch the left leg forward, heel on the ground and toes flexed. Stretch your arms forward, parallel to the ground, hands in fists, thumbs pointing up. Maintain the arms parallel to the ground and inhale as you stretch forward from the hips, exhale as you lean backward. Continue for **30 seconds**. Switch legs and repeat the exercise with the right leg stretched forward for **30 seconds**. Breathe powerfully.
It is common to see the arms drop on the forward motion and lift on the backward motion.

---

1 Authors' Note: For those who are older, it is good to pull the toes toward oneself during the exercise, so that the muscles are active and the joints will be better protected. Start by bringing the tailbone, navel and Heart Center aligned.

→ continue on next page

KUNDALINI YOGA FOR SELF-CARE AND CAREGIVERS

8) PELVIC LIFTS[1].

Lie on the back with the knees bent. Place the soles of the feet hip-width apart flat on the ground, heels at the buttocks. Grasp the ankles. Inhale and lift the pelvis up; exhale and lower the pelvis down to the ground. Continue for **1-3 minutes**.

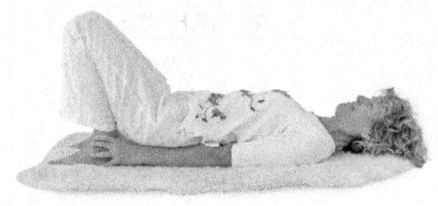

9) MODIFIED CAT-COW[2].

Come onto your hands and knees in Cow Pose, with knees directly under the hips and arms straight, palms flat on the ground directly under the shoulders. Arch the spine downward, lowering the abdomen and lifting the sternum and chin. Extend the right leg back and raise it as high as possible with pointed toes on the inhale. Round the spine up toward the ceiling, bring the chin toward the chest and pull the right knee to the forehead on the exhale. Do not over-extend. Continue for **1-3 minutes**. Switch legs and continue for **1-3 minutes**. Breathe powerfully.

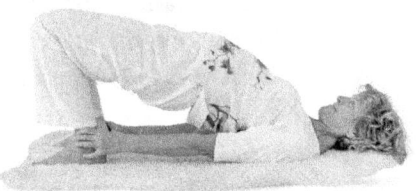

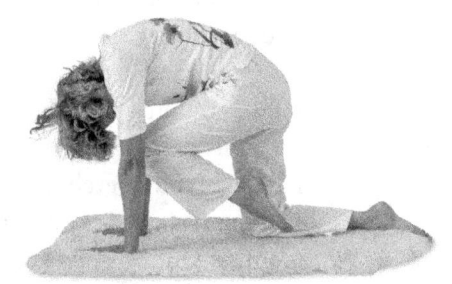

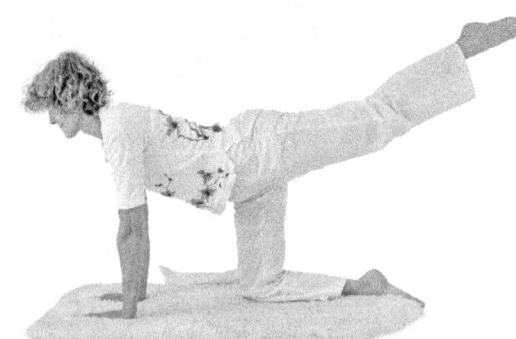

---

1 Authors' Note: Variation: If necessary, use a cork block to maintain the space between the knees. If you cannot grab your ankles, place the arms next to your hips with the palms down. You can use the underarms to lift yourself off the ground when pushing the pelvis upward.

2 Authors' Note: While on the mat, make sure that your hands are placed exactly under your shoulders, and keep your elbows straight. If you have problems in your wrist, consider doing the exercise making fists with your hands.

8) PELVIC LIFTS.

Remain seated in the middle of the chair with the feet next to each other. Grasp the edges of the chair or place the forearms on the armrests. Breathe in. Push the feet and knees together and contract the pelvic floor muscles. Lift the pelvis slightly off the chair if possible, or visualize it. Open the chest. Breathe out, slowly lower the pelvis and relax. Repeat in a slow rhythm for **1 minute**.

9) MODIFIED CAT-COW[2].

Sit actively at the front of the chair with a straight spine. Exhale, round the back and bring the right knee toward the body. Inhale, stretch your back, open your chest, and slide the right foot under the chair. Continue for **1 minute**, then change to the other leg. Continue for **1 minute**.

---

2 When performing this adaptation, use caution and be aware of your sense of balance and limitations. You can always opt to visualize the exercise when you don't feel confident about what the movement entails to you and your body. [Editor's Note]

10) KIDNEY STRETCH.

Sit on the heels in Rock Pose, bend forward and place the forearms on the ground in front of the knees with the palms together with the thumbs pointing up. Inhale and stretch forward over the palms, exhale and return to the initial position. Keep the chin up and body parallel to the ground creating a pressure on the lower back. Continue for **1-3 minutes**.

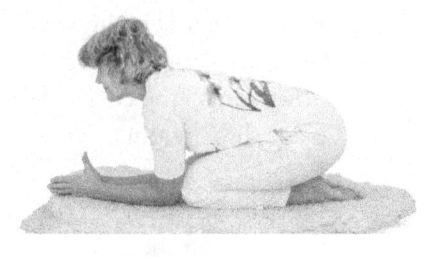
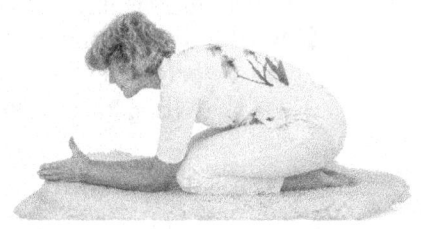

11) BACK ROLLS[3].

Lay on the back. Pull the knees into the chest, wrap the arms around the front of the legs just below the knees. Tuck the chin into the chest with the nose between the knees. Roll back and forth on your spine for **1-3 minutes**.

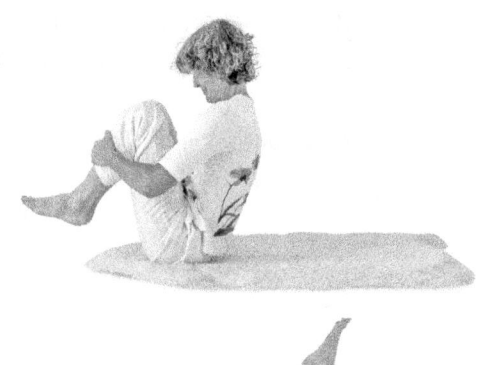
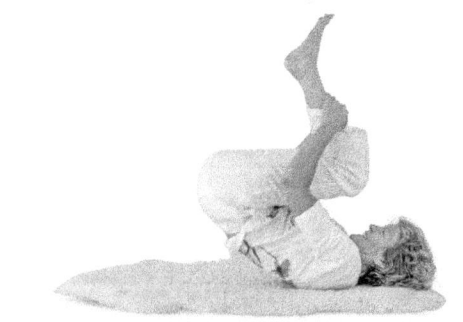

---

3 Authors' Note: You can place an extra blanket or mat under your back to protect the spine.

→ continue on next page

10) KIDNEY STRETCH.

Remain seated and place your elbows on the knees, forearms parallel to the ground and press the palms together with the thumbs pointing upward. Breathe in and move the upper body forward over your hands, breathe out and move backward while keeping the spine straight and chin up, creating a pressure on the lower back. Continue for **1 minute**.

11) BACK ROLLS[3].

Remain seated, grab the knees and bend slightly forward with a round back. Rock forward and backward as much as possible keeping the back rounded. The feet may come off the ground. Continue for **1 minute**.

---

3 When performing this adaptation, use caution and be aware of your sense of balance and your limitations. You can always opt to visualize the exercise when you don't feel confident about what the movement entails to you and your body. [Editor's Note]

→ continue on next page

12) RELAXATION.

Lie down on the back in Corpse Pose and relax for one full hour. It is recommended to drink a glass of water.

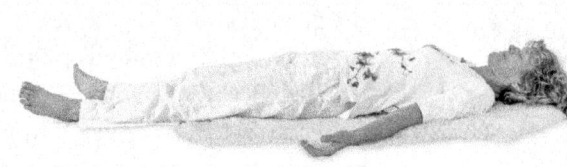

Comments: Our energy can be flowing, we can be eating well, sleeping enough, but if our adrenals fail, it is hard to keep up. We get tired and snappy. Glandular balance and, in particular, strong adrenals and kidneys are important to have that extra edge, to control anger and hypoglycemia. Strong adrenals and kidneys promote healthy heart function.

12) RELAXATION.

Sit with the feet comfortably apart on the ground and connect with the earth. Your back is against the seat back with the lower spine well-supported. Relax the hands on the upper legs, palms up. It is recommended to drink a glass of water before relaxing for an hour.

Comments: Our energy can be flowing, we can be eating well, sleeping enough, but if our adrenals fail, it is hard to keep up. We get tired and snappy. Glandular balance and, in particular, strong adrenals and kidneys are important to have that extra edge, to control anger and hypoglycemia. Strong adrenals and kidneys promote healthy heart function.

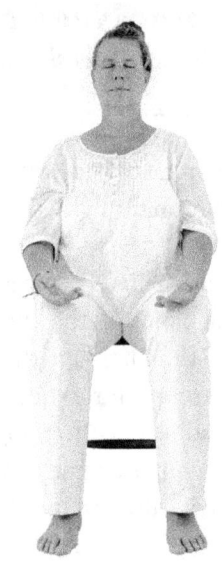

5.3 Antar Naad Mudra - Kabadshe Meditation
Originally published in the Aquarian Teacher Yoga Manual

Sit in Easy Pose with a straight spine and a light Neck Lock.

Mudra: Extend the arms with the hands on the knees. Touch the thumb tips to the tips of the Mercury (little) fingers in Buddhi Mudra. The other fingers are relaxed straight. Become completely still, physically and mentally, like a calm ocean. If listening to a recording of the mantra, listen to the chant for a minute, feeling its rhythm in every cell. Then begin to chant with it.

**Mantra: SAA RAY SAA SAA, SAA RAY SAA SAA, SAA RAY SAA SAA, SAA RUNG
HAR RAY HAR HAR, HAR RAY HAR HAR, HAR RAY HAR HAR, HAR RUNG**

Time: 11-31 minutes.

Comments: Antar Naad Mudra is the meditation that opens up the chakras for the full effect of any other mantra. It is a sensitizing meditation for the impact of the inner sound current. It is the base of all mantras. The original practice of mastery in mantra required that you master this before any other mantra practice. The esoteric structure of the mantra is coded in the qualities that each of the sounds represents, and the rhythm that weaves them together into a coherent and powerful effect. **SAA** means the Infinite, the totality, God. It is the element of ether. It initiates and contains all other effects. It is subtle and beyond. **HAR** is the creativity of the earth. It is a dense element. It is the power of manifestation, the tangible, the personal. These sounds are woven together then projected through the sound of **UNG** or complete totality, like the original sound **AUM** or **ONG**. This meditation is said to bring protection, prosperity, and creativity.

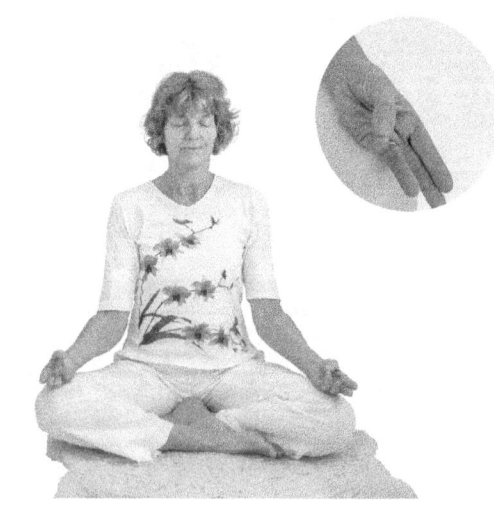

ON THE CHAIR

Sit comfortably in a chair with the weight of both feet resting evenly on the ground, with a straight spine, and a light Neck Lock.

Practice as described on the side.

Time: Start with **5 minutes** and slowly build up to **11 minutes**.

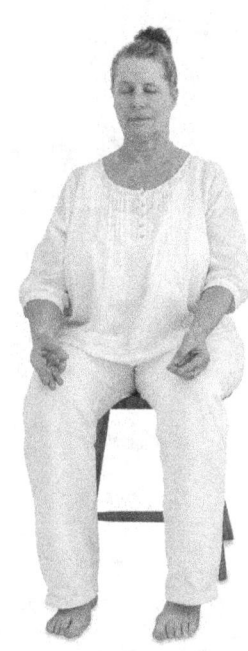
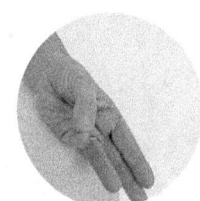

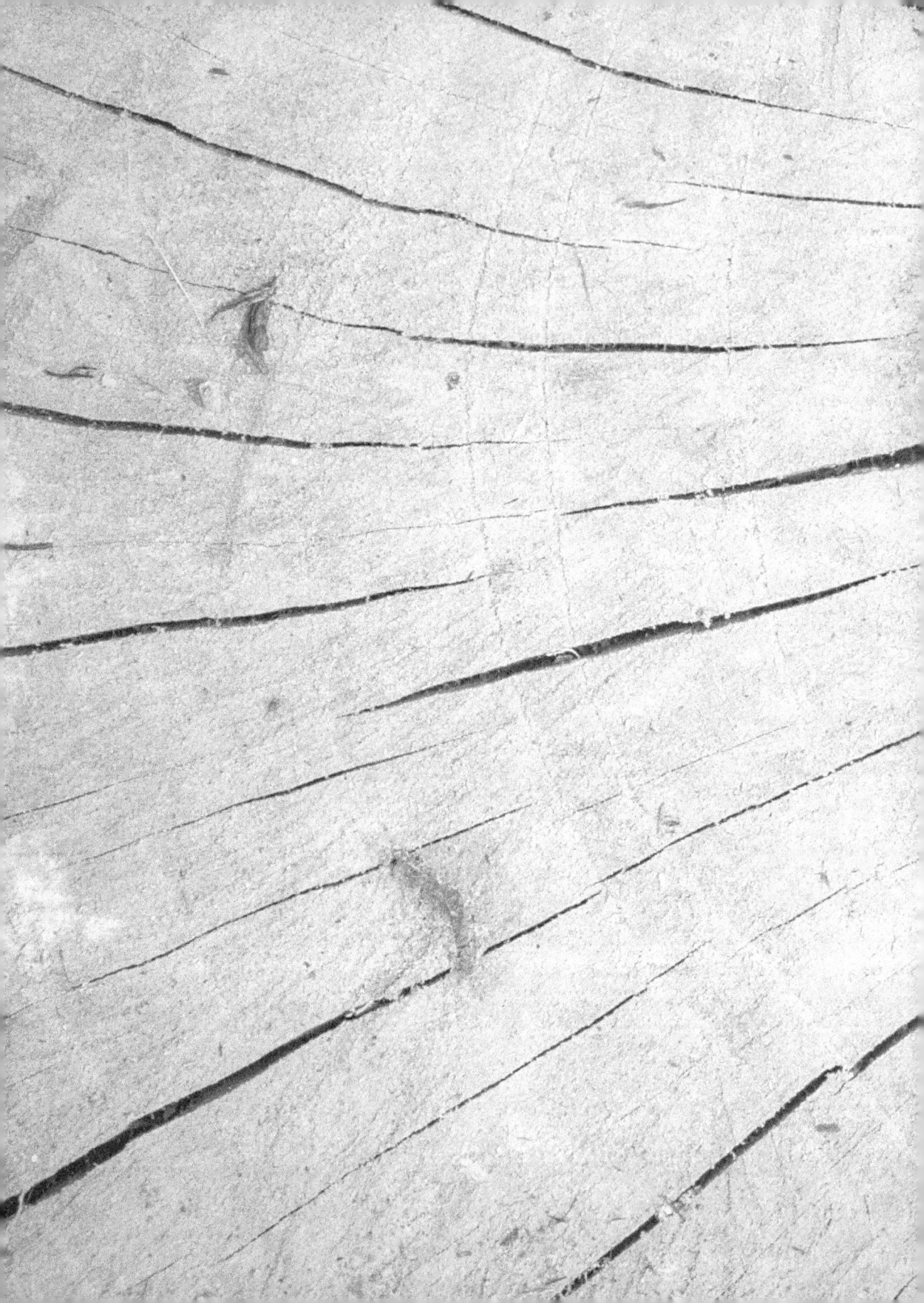

CHAPTER 6
Self-Esteem

—

Real happiness is when you are you, and you are powerful within you. It is your power in you, which is useful and powerful, and it is understood by others.

— YOGI BHAJAN, NOVEMBER 26, 1989

In this chapter you will work on the third chakra also known as Manipura, which is situated in the Navel Point area, near the solar plexus. It is connected to your will and ego, but it is also linked to commitment and the courage to live from quiet willpower and self-esteem. The third chakra is your center of personal power and the region of healthy identity and the ability to manifest. Having a strong third chakra also means good health and a strong constitution. Food and impressions are digested in the area of the third chakra, the physical center of the body, the location of the stomach, and digestive system. This chakra is related to inner balance and your sense of humor.

The third chakra's motto is: *I connect myself to action.* Yellow is the color associated with this chakra. The subtle perception is vision. The element is fire. Organs associated with this chakra are the liver, gallbladder, pancreas, spleen, the stomach, and digestive system.

When out of balance, this chakra's dysfunction can manifest as oppression, lack of power, feeling weak, anger, greed, shame, procrastination, getting carried away. It can be experienced as denying one's own wishes and emotions. In the physical body, problems with the digestion, the liver, the gallbladder and the pancreas can all be related to a weak third chakra.

In terms of childhood development, a child generally discovers that they have a will around the age of 1.5 years old, when the autonomy phase begins. In this phase the third chakra develops and opens. This phase is often a considerable challenge for parents. They have to teach their children that their will is important, but that it also needs to coexist with their surroundings. The child should feel free to express itself, and should be allowed to get frustrated in a healthy way. Parents need to offer consistent support, so that their child can grow up to be a peaceful warrior rather than a depressive person.

What affects the third chakra: all exercises that train the abdominal muscles or that work on the navel plexus and Navel point; exercises that increase the fire energy like Breath of Fire; exercises that work in the area of the solar plexus such as Diaphragm Lock.

The breath, kriya, and meditation practices listed below aid in the process of becoming aware of your ego, your identity (what you stand for), the fire element, your power and limitations, but also your will to survive. The mantras and chanting develop courage and fearlessness.

The breath practice *Self-Care Breath* is a healing breath that increases inner energy and strength, and cleanses the body. The *Kriya to Take Away Fear and Sadness* helps you in the release of anger, fear, and sorrow. The kriya utilizes the *Har* mantra; the physical action of quickly pulling in the Navel Point in chanting this mantra clearly engages the navel energy. The Har mantra affects the Navel Point, empowers and develops willpower. The kriya also works directly on the stomach, which is considered to be connected to balancing other body systems.

The Har Har Mukande mantra, which appears in both the *Kriya to Take Away Fear and Sadness* and the *Meditation for the Third Chakra*, plays a role in liberation and letting go of your sorrow. "Mukande" means liberator. *Chattr Chakkr Vartee* is a mantra used to overcome fear and phobias. It is a mantra to experience victory.

The *Meditation for the Third Chakra* provides determination and strong nerves. In this meditation the mantra *Humee Hum Brahm Hum* means that we carry the spirit of the divine, that the divine is present in us. It confirms the identity in its true reality.

6.1 Self-Care Breath: Healing Pranayam

Originally published in Serving the Infinite - Transformation Vol. 2

Sit in Easy Pose with a straight spine and a light Neck Lock.

Mudra: Place the hands crossed on the Heart Center, right over left.

Eye Focus: Closed.

Breath: Breathe a steady, powerful Cannon Breath. Breath of Fire through a firm "O" mouth. The pressure of the breath is in the cheeks and over the tongue, though there should be no bulging of the cheeks.

Mental Focus: Sense the area under the palms. Let the mind focus on the "O" mouth and shape the breath into a ring.

Time: 5 minutes.

To End: Inhale, suspend the breath, relax the mouth, mentally repeat: "I am beautiful, I am innocent, I am innocent, I am beautiful," exhale through the nose. Repeat **4 more times**.

Comments: Self-care breath increases inner energy and strength, boosts the immune system, and cleanses the body.

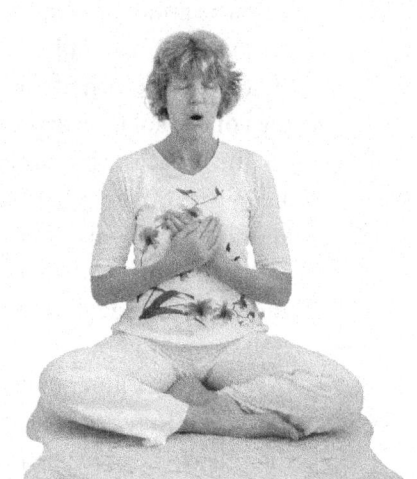

ON THE CHAIR

Sit comfortably in a chair with the weight of both feet resting evenly on the ground, with a straight spine, and a light Neck Lock.

Practice as described on the side.

Time: Start with **1 minute** and gradually increase the time to **5 minutes**.

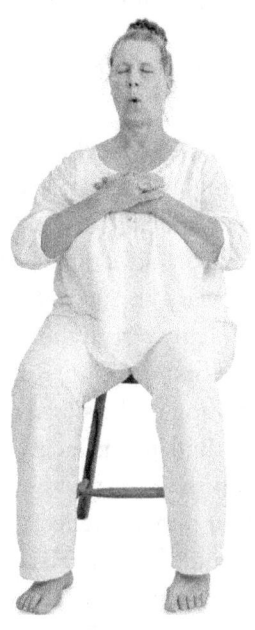

6.2 Kriya to Take Away Fear and Sadness
May 8, 1985

There are no breaks between exercises.

1) ELBOW STRETCH.
Sit in Easy Pose with a straight spine and a light Neck Lock. Bend the elbows bringing the hands near the shoulders, palms facing forward. With a quick motion like a punch, shoot the arms forward and up to a 60-degree angle. Quickly return the arms and hands to the first position. Repeat the outward motion to the sides, parallel to the ground, palms facing down, and quickly return to the first position. Create a four part sequence, drawing the navel in and chanting **HAR** with the tip of the tongue on each movement. Move rhythmically, **3 seconds** per complete cycle. Continue for **3 ½ minutes**.
The outward motions are powerful to stretch the elbow.

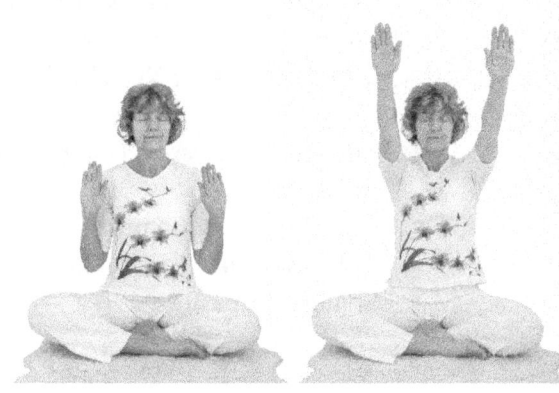

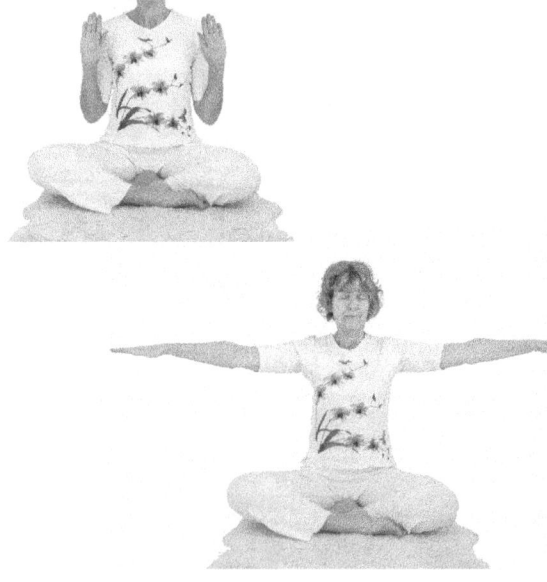

→ continue on next page

ON THE CHAIR

1) ELBOW STRETCH.
Sit in a chair, feet hip-width apart and even weight on both feet with a straight spine, and a light Neck Lock. Bend the elbows bringing the hands near the shoulders, palms forward. With a quick motion, shoot the arms forward and up at a 60-degree angle. Quickly return the arms and hands to the first position. Repeat the outward motion to the sides, arms parallel to the ground, palms facing down and quickly return to the first position. Create a four part sequence, drawing the navel in and chanting **HAR** with the tip of the tongue on each movement. Move rhythmically, 3 seconds per complete cycle. Continue for **1 minute and 45 seconds**.
The outward motions are powerful to stretch the elbow.

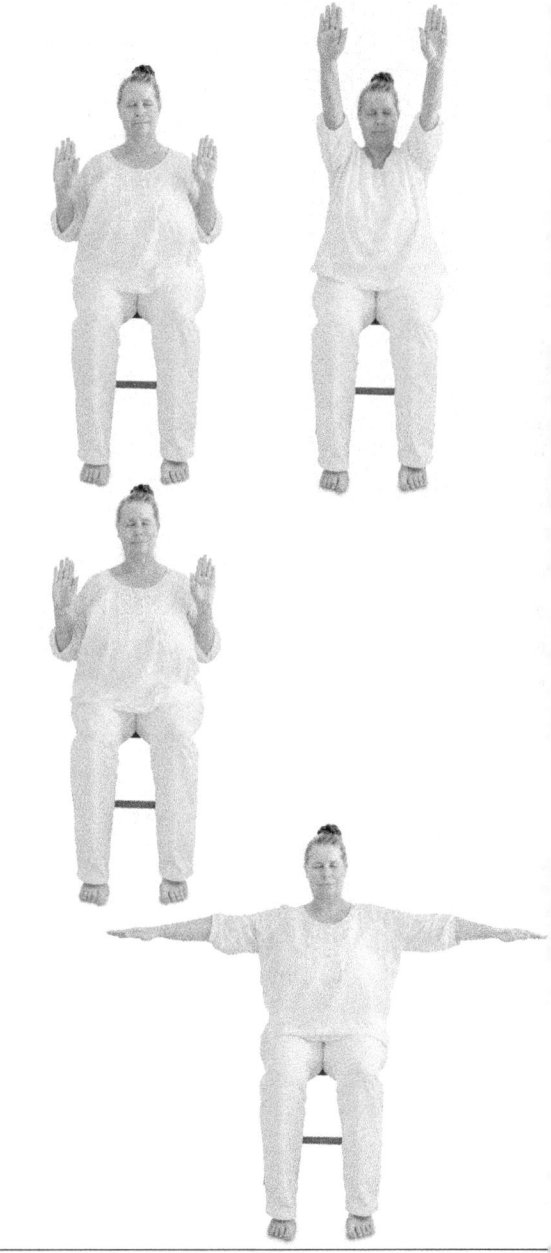

→ continue on next page

2) ELBOW STRETCH WITH TONGUE OUT. Remain in Easy Pose and repeat exercise 1 with the tongue extended out of the mouth, still chanting **HAR** at each position. Punch with the force of your anger in the same rhythm. Continue for **2 ½ minutes**.

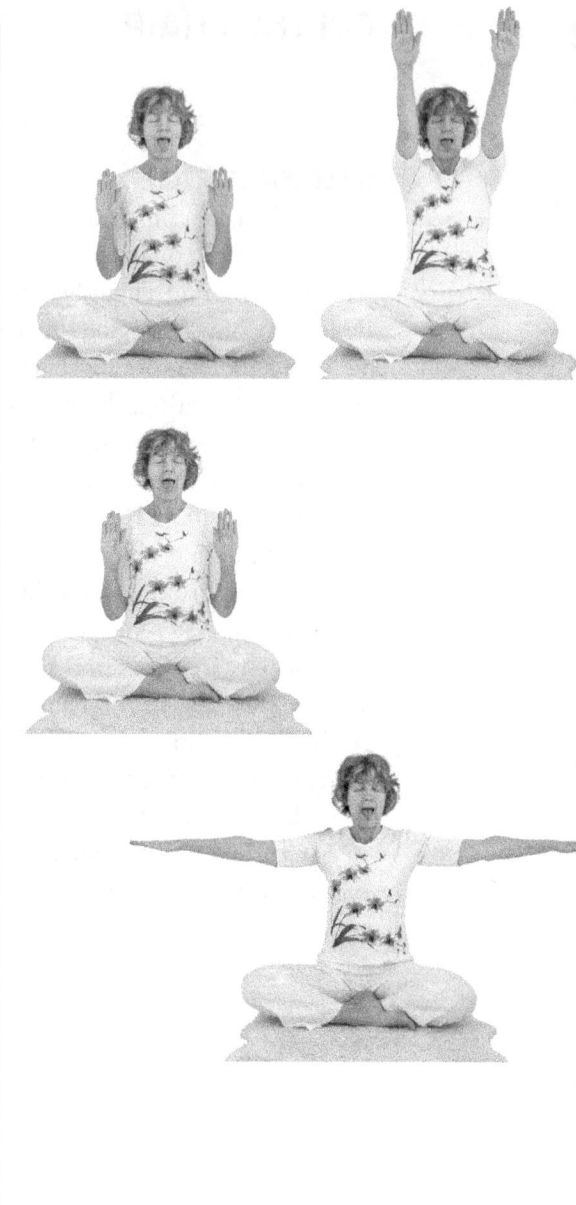

→ continue on next page

2) ELBOW STRETCH WITH TONGUE OUT.

Repeat exercise 1 with the tongue extended out of the mouth, still chanting **HAR** with each movement. Push out with the force of your anger in the same rhythm. Continue for **1 minute and 15 seconds**.

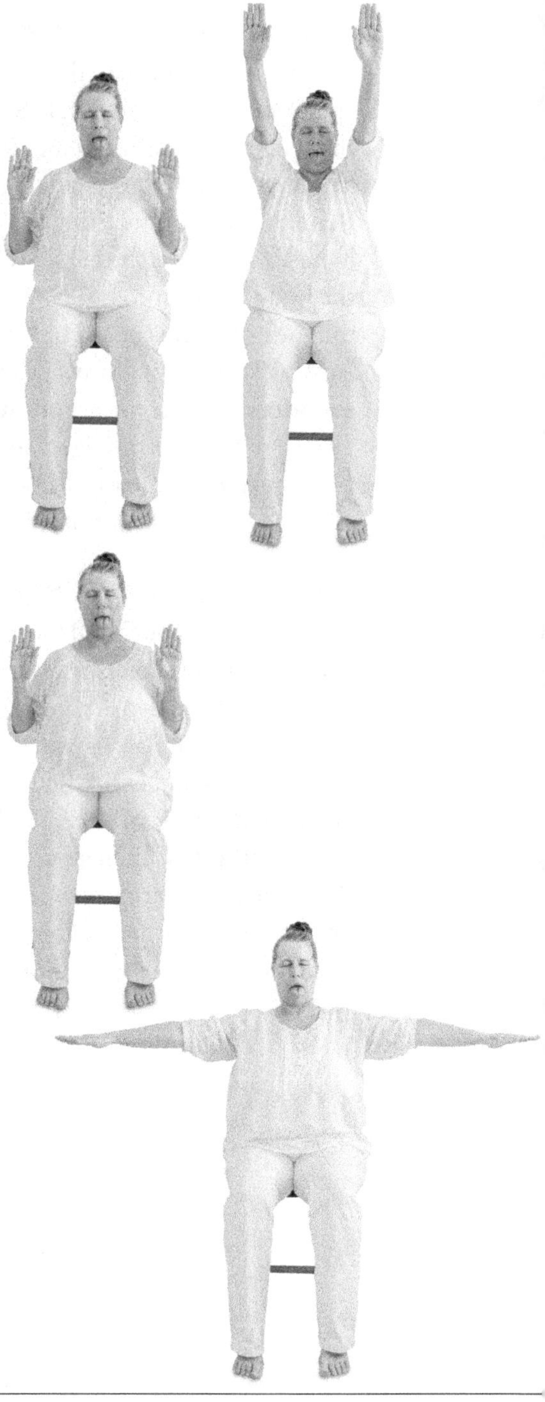

→ continue on next page

3) SPINAL TWIST VARIATION.

Remain in Easy Pose with a straight spine and a light Neck Lock. Stretch the arms to the sides at shoulder height with the palms facing forward. Bend the elbows and bring the hands in fists near the ears. Twist the body from left to right. With the tongue extended, chant **HAR** with each twist. Twist to both sides per **1 second**. Continue for **1 ½ minutes**. *This exercise makes the chest more flexible and massages the heart area, allowing sorrow to be released.*

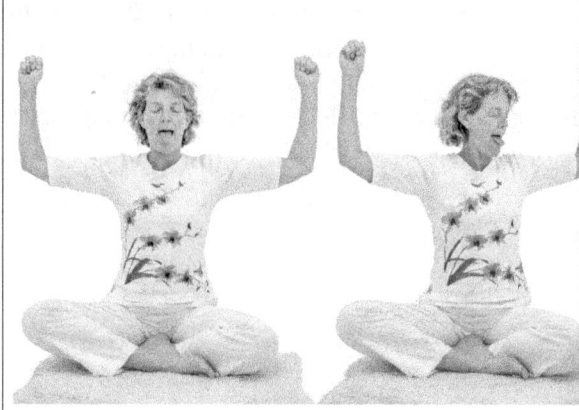

4) BABY POSE WITH CHANTING.

Sit on the heels and bend forward with the forehead on the ground and the arms at the sides of the body with palms up in Baby Pose. Relax the shoulders and entire body and chant **HAR HAR MUKANDAY** for **9 ½ minutes**. Then sit up in Easy Pose, extend the arms forward and up at a 60-degree angle. Continue to chant for another **1 ½ minutes**.

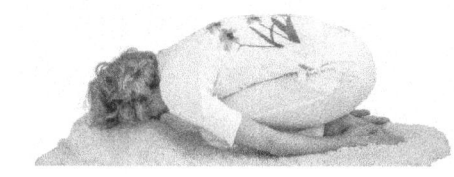

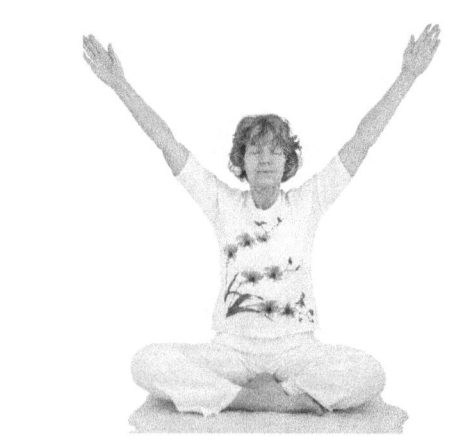

3) SPINAL TWIST VARIATION.
Remain seated with a straight spine and the feet hip-width apart. Stretch the arms to the sides at shoulder height with the palms facing forward. Bend the elbows and bring the hands in fists near the ears. Twist the body, left to right. With the tongue extended, chant **HAR** with each twist. Twist to both sides per **1 second**. Continue for **1 minute**. *This exercise makes the chest more flexible and massages the heart area, allowing sorrow to be released.*

4) BABY POSE WITH CHANTING.
Remain seated with the feet a bit further apart. Place the forearms on the thighs or on the armrests. Make fists, bend the upper body forward and rest your forehead on your fists. You can also place your arms on a table. Relax, and feel sleepy while chanting: **HAR HAR MUKANDAY**. Continue for **4 minutes and 45 seconds**. Then gently sit up straight, stretch the arms up at a 60-degree angle. In case of shoulder conditions, place the hands next to the shoulders. Continue chanting **HAR HAR MUKANDAY** for **1 more minute**. *Do not put the head lower than the heart in case of high blood pressure or heart problems, but rest your head on a pillow or blanket. Baby Pose helps you to feel like a child again, allowing you to start over. This exercise helps to turn inward and come to yourself.*

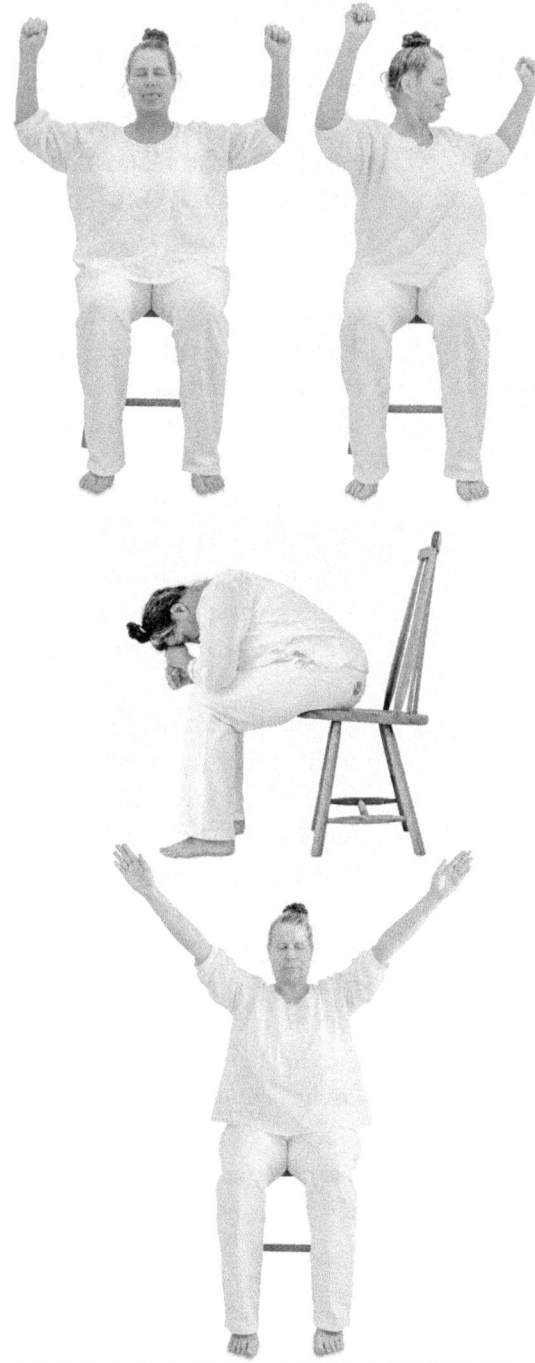

KUNDALINI YOGA FOR SELF-CARE AND CAREGIVERS

5) MEDITATE.

Remain in Easy Pose, allow your head to hang, let your shoulders drop and feel very sad and tired. Silently meditate on the mantra **CHATTR CHAKKR VARTEE.** (The last four lines of Jaap Sahib. In the original class, a recording by Kulwant Singh was played.) Continue for **6 minutes**. Then sit up straight with the hands in your lap, and meditate with the music for **3 more minutes**.
TO END: Inhale, suspend the breath for **30 seconds**, exhale. Repeat **3 more times**.
It doesn't matter how much sorrow there is, this exercise and mantra support you to have courage and keep up.

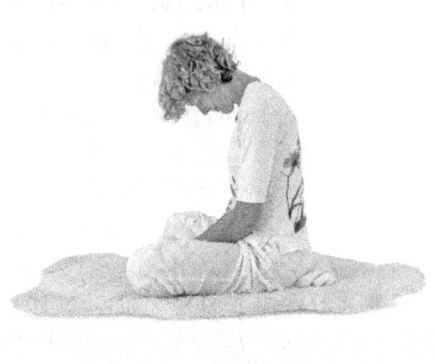

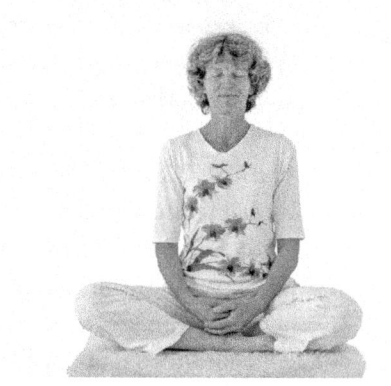

Comments: The body's entire creative sensitivity is in the stomach. The stomach stimulates the brain to coordinate the entire system. Both the heart and brain are subject to the stomach. When ancient yogis learned this fact, they developed a whole science of fasting and food combining. The elbow area controls the stomach and this yoga set opens up the elbow to work on the stomach. Practicing this set can be beneficial for the stomach and remove sadness and fear from your personality.

5) MEDITATE.
Remain seated, allow your head to hang, let the shoulders drop and feel very sad and tired. Silently meditate on the mantra **CHATTR CHAKKR VARTEE**. (The last four lines of Jaap Sahib. In the original class, a recording by Kulwant Singh was played.) Continue for **3 minutes**. Then sit up straight with your hands in your lap, continue to meditate on the music for **1 more minute**.
TO END: Inhale, suspend the breath as long as comfortable, exhale. Repeat **3 more times**.
It doesn't matter how much sorrow there is, this exercise and mantra support you to have courage and keep up.

Comments: The body's entire creative sensitivity is in the stomach. The stomach stimulates the brain to coordinate the entire system. Both the heart and brain are subject to the stomach. When ancient yogis learned this fact, they developed a whole science of fasting and food combining. The elbow area controls the stomach and this yoga set opens up the elbow to work on the stomach. Practicing this set can be beneficial for the stomach and remove sadness and fear from your personality.

Authors' Recommendation: Deep relaxation. Sit in the back of the chair, so that the lower back is fully supported. Let the hands rest in the lap with the palms open and upward. Shut your eyes and relax for **11 minutes**.

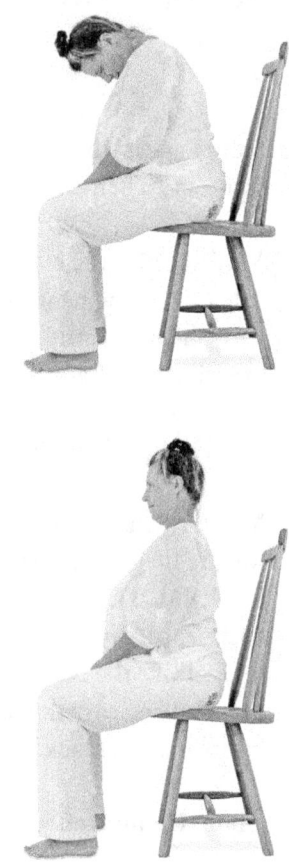

6.3 Meditation for the Third Chakra
February 5 & 6, 1991

Sit in Easy Pose with a straight spine and a light Neck Lock.

Mudra: With the elbows relaxed at the sides, bring the hands into Prayer Pose with all parts of the palms touching and pressing together with equal force.

Eye Focus: Tip of the Nose.

Mantra: Chant with the tip of the tongue the mantra **HUMME HUM, BRAHM HUM**[1]. As you chant each word, simultaneously pull in and release the Navel Point, and press and release the hands. The entire mantra takes 3 seconds.

Time: 11 minutes (maximum).

To End: Inhale and suspend the breath, pull in on the navel and press the tip of the tongue against the roof of the mouth. Suspend the breath for **15 seconds** and exhale. Repeat the sequence for **2 more times**. Relax.

Comments: The hand press is a compression, like the beat of the heart. When this meditation has been perfected in this form, it may be practiced with the Root Lock applied.

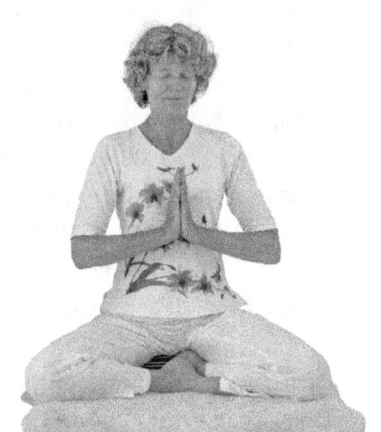

---

1 Authors' Note: The mantra Humee Hum, Brahm Hum means that we hold the spirit of the divine, that the divine is present in us. It confirms the identity in its true reality.

ON THE CHAIR

Sit comfortably in a chair with the weight of both feet resting evenly on the ground, with a straight spine, and a light Neck Lock.

Practice as described on the side.

Time: Start with **3 minutes** and gradually build up to a maximum of **11 minutes**.

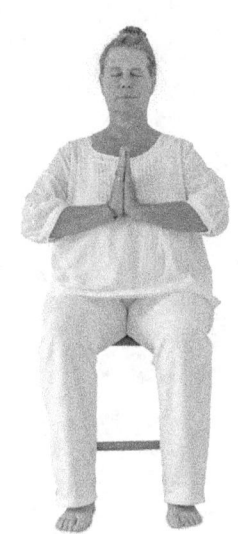

CHAPTER 7
Awareness

—

Value yourself as God's will. Then let your will value yourself as a God will.

— YOGI BHAJAN, JULY 6, 1994

This chapter will focus on the fourth chakra, the Anahata or the Heart Center. Before delving deeper into the heart chakra, it is important to understand that it's a transitional point where animal or instinctive energy transforms into higher awareness. The energy released by the lower chakras is used to cultivate awareness in the fourth chakra. An awakening then occurs in the upper chakras, the fifth through seventh chakras.

The lower three chakras are the foundation of your life, your driving force, and your instinct. Because the themes of these chakras are subconscious, acting from the expression of the lower chakras feels natural.

Working on yourself in subtle ways allows you to become aware of the energy of these chakras and then transform it. Yoga, meditation, and therapy can all help you to balance these themes from the lower three chakras and the subconscious energy held there. The fourth chakra serves as a gateway between the lower and upper chakras.

The fourth chakra is located in the center of the chest, near the heart. It is associated with love, compassion, and empathy, as well as with the recognition and understanding of others' virtues. This chakra represents the beginning of consciousness, awareness and subtlety. This lesson will focus on your gut instinct and breath, as well as self-love and love.

This chakras' motto is: *I love and I empathize*. Green is the color associated with this chakra. The element is air. The subtle perception is touch. The organs for the fourth chakra include the heart, lungs, and thymus gland.

Chakra imbalances can manifest as fear of losing love, and thus no longer being connected with love; dependence on love, fear of rejection, being easily hurt, attachment, helpers syndrome, and heartlessness. The heart chakra deals with the feelings of sorrow and fear. In the physical body, problems with the heart, lungs, and blood pressure can be related to a weak fourth chakra.

In terms of childhood development, during the time of puberty the heart chakra opens. Until that time, a child lives (in a natural and healthy manner) self-absorbed and without introspection. At this age stage, you see your parents as individuals with peculiarities and faults. You observe these peculiarities and judge them. At puberty, the learning task is to unconditionally share the essence of life with yourself and others. For this to happen compassion and surrender are required.

What affects the fourth chakra: Arm exercises, upper body twisting exercises, and chest opening exercises are all examples of heart and lung exercises; all breath exercises; all chanting. Any exercises that promote love, compassion and forgiveness. The fourth chakra is strengthened when you are reassured and comforted, and when you walk, dance, and sing.

The first kriya, called the *Kriya for Expanding Lung Capacity* is an advanced exercise that improves your lung and breath capacity, while also being beneficial for the heart. The *Kriya to Open the Heart Center* focuses on opening the Heart Center, so you can observe love and self-love. This kriya also relaxes the mind, allowing you to be more present and experience clarity with your feelings. The *Meditation for a Calm Heart*, a breath-focused meditation, promotes a calm and peaceful heart. This stillness and peace in the Heart Center is the hallmark of the balanced fourth chakra.

7.1 Kriya for Expanding Lung Capacity
Originally published in Sadhana Guidelines

1) LUNG ENERGIZER.
Sit in Easy Pose with a straight spine and a light Neck Lock. Stretch the arms out to the sides at shoulder level. Raise the forearms perpendicular to the ground. Bend the wrists back, the fingers point to the sides, and palms face up. Hold for **1 minute**.
TO END: Inhale deeply, suspend the breath for **10 seconds**, exhale. Repeat **3 more times**. On the third exhale, suspend the breath out and apply Root Lock. Inhale, suspend the breath briefly, and exhale.

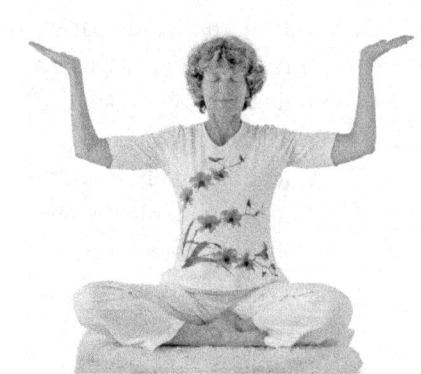

2) LONG DEEP BREATH.
Remain in Easy Pose with the hands relaxed in the lap in Venus Lock. Begin Long Deep Breathing for **10 minutes**. With each inhalation, expand the ribcage to fully inhale. Immediately begin Exercise 3. *Concentrate firmly at the Third Eye Point to maintain a balanced breath.*

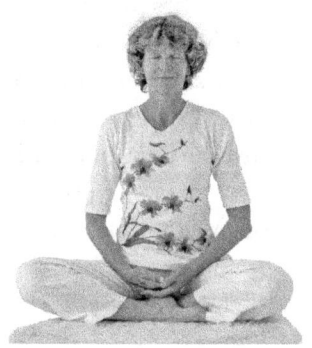

→ continue on next page

ON THE CHAIR

1) LUNG ENERGIZE.
Sit in a chair, feet hip-width apart and even weight on both feet with a straight spine, and a light Neck Lock. Stretch the arms out to the sides at shoulder level. Raise the forearms perpendicular to the ground. Bend the wrists, fingers point to the sides and palms face up. Hold for **1 minute**. TO END: Inhale deeply, suspend the breath for **10 seconds**, exhale. Repeat **3 more times**. On the third exhale, suspend the breath out and apply Root Lock. Inhale, suspend the breath briefly, and exhale.

2) LONG DEEP BREATH.
Remain seated with a straight spine. Hands relaxed in the lap in Venus Lock. Begin Long Deep Breathing for **5 minutes**. With each inhalation, expand the ribcage to fully inhale. *Concentrate firmly at the Third Eye Point to maintain a balanced breath.*

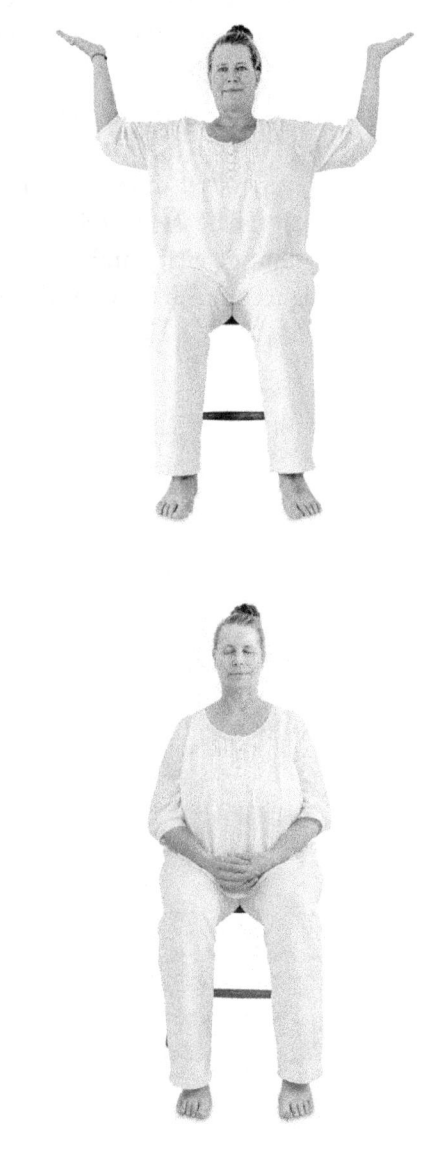

→ continue on next page

3) PRAANA BALANCE.

Sit with the legs extended with the feet together. Bend forward from the hips and hold the toes. Inhale, exhale, suspend the breath out while pumping the navel as long as you can comfortably suspend the breath out. Repeat **2 more times**.

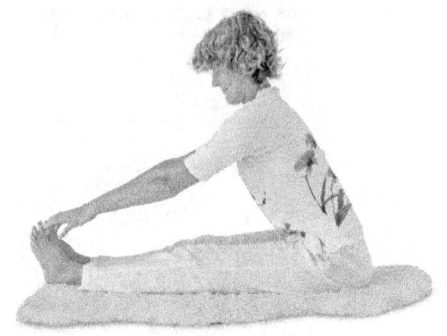

Comments: Exercise 1 energizes the lungs and heart. Exercise 2 expands the lung capacity, and Exercise 3 balances and distributes the praana.

3) PRAANA BALANCE.

Remain seated, stretch your left leg forward with the foot resting on the heel, toes flexed. The right foot stays flat on the ground. Bend forward from the hips with the back stretched and grasp the stretched leg. Inhale, exhale, suspend the breath out while pumping your belly for as long as you can comfortably suspend the breath out. Repeat the exercise with an outstretched right leg.

Comments: Exercise 1 energizes the lungs and heart. Exercise 2 expands the lung capacity, and Exercise 3 balances and distributes the praana.

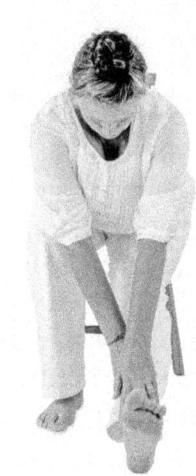

7.2 Kriya to Open the Heart Center
Originally published in Serving the Infinite - Transformation Vol. 2

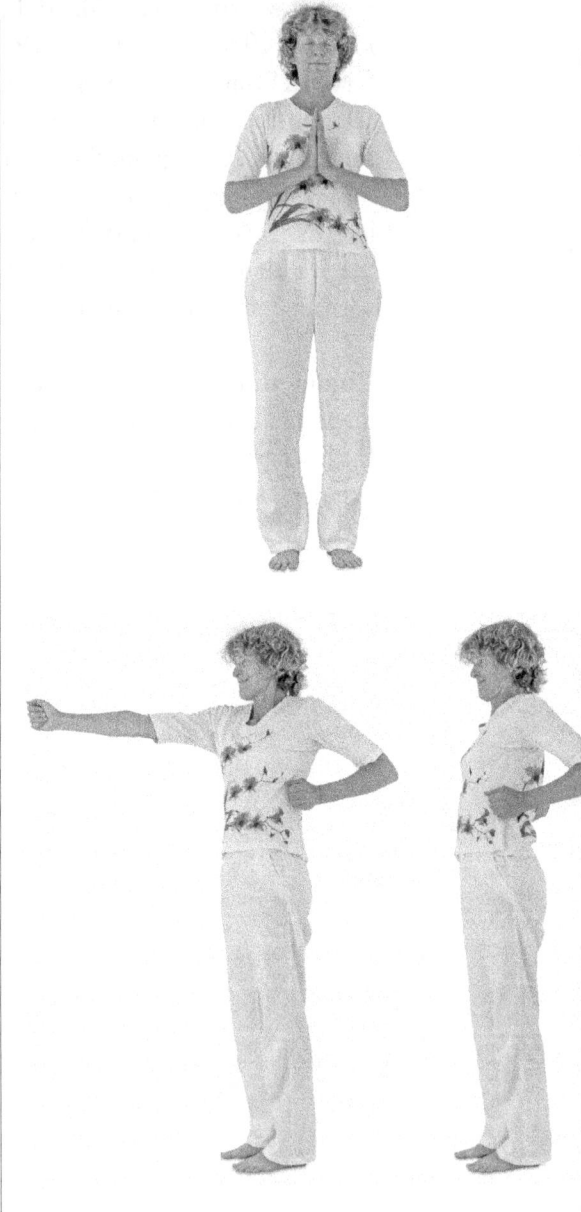

1) PRAYER POSE WITH BREATH OF FIRE.
Stand with a straight spine and a light Neck Lock. Press the hands together at the Heart Center in Prayer Pose. Continue for **3 minutes** with Breath of Fire.
TO END: Inhale, suspend the breath briefly, and exhale.

2) PISTON PUNCHING.
Remain standing or sit in Easy Pose with a straight spine and a light Neck Lock. The eyes are open and gaze at the horizon. Make fists with the palms facing each other. Alternately, punch forward with your left and right fists. Together the hands create a piston-like motion with one arm pulling back and the other arm punching forward. The hands do not turn or twist. Punch rapidly, exhaling with each punch, so the breath becomes like Breath of Fire. Continue for **3 minutes**.
TO END: Inhale, draw both elbows back, tighten the fists, apply Root Lock, and suspend the breath for **5 seconds**, exhale, and relax.

→ continue on next page

ON THE CHAIR

1) PRAYER POSE WITH BREATH OF FIRE.
Sit in a chair, feet hip-width apart and even weight on both feet with a straight spine and a light Neck Lock. Connect with the earth under your feet. Press the hands together at the center of the chest in Prayer Pose. Continue for **1 minute** with Breath of Fire.
TO END: Inhale, suspend the breath briefly, exhale, and relax.

2) PISTON PUNCHING.
Remain seated with a straight spine. The eyes open and gaze at the horizon. Make fists with the palms facing each other. Pull both elbows backward. Alternatingly, punch forward with your left and right fists. Together the hands create a piston-like motion with one arm pulling back and the other arm punching forward. The hands do not turn or twist. Punch rapidly, exhaling with each punch, so the breath becomes like Breath of Fire. Continue for **1 minute**.
TO END: Inhale, draw both elbows back, tighten the fists, apply Root Lock, and suspend the breath for **5 seconds**, exhale, and relax.

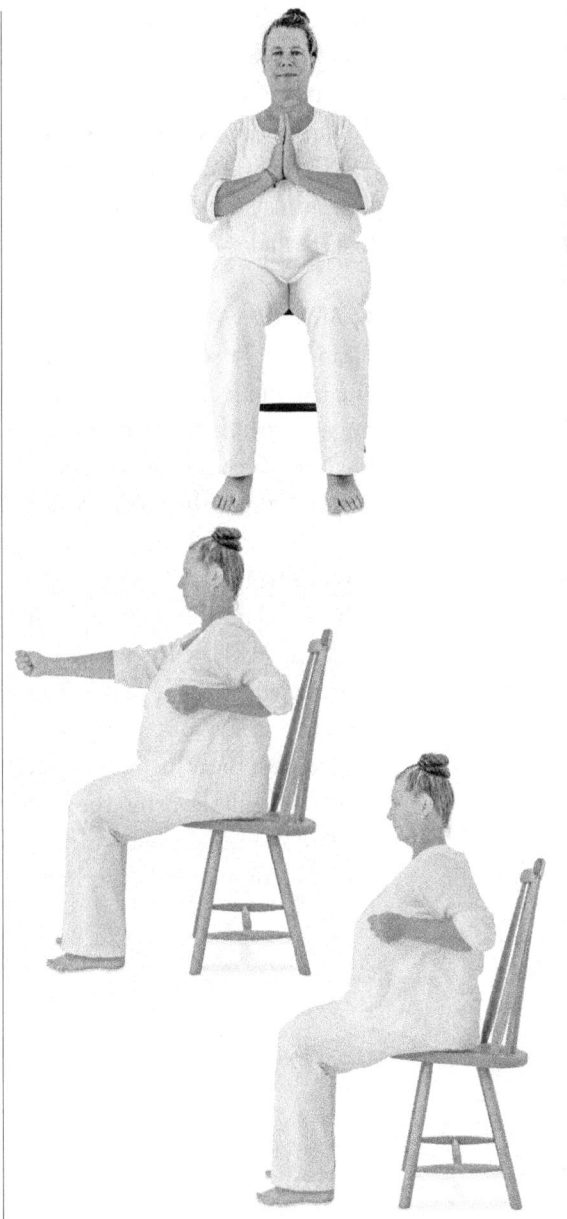

→ continue on next page

3) BACKWARD ARMS CIRCLES.

Stand with a straight spine and a light Neck Lock. Stretch the arms out to the sides, and move both arms together in large backward circles. Inhale as they come forward and up, and exhale as they go back and down. Continue for **2 minutes**.
TO END: Inhale and stretch both arms straight up over your head, exhale, and relax.

4) ARM PUMP VARIATION.

Sit in Easy Pose with a straight spine and a light Neck Lock. Interlace your fingers with the thumb tips touching. Position the hands 4-6 inches (10-15 cm) in front of the chest, palms facing down. Elbows are out to the sides with the forearms parallel to the ground. Inhale and lift the arms and hands up to the level of the throat. Exhale and lower them to the level of the navel. Create a steady pumping motion for **3 minutes**. Breathe powerfully.
TO END: Inhale, bring the hands to the level of the heart, suspend the breath for 10 seconds, exhale, and relax.

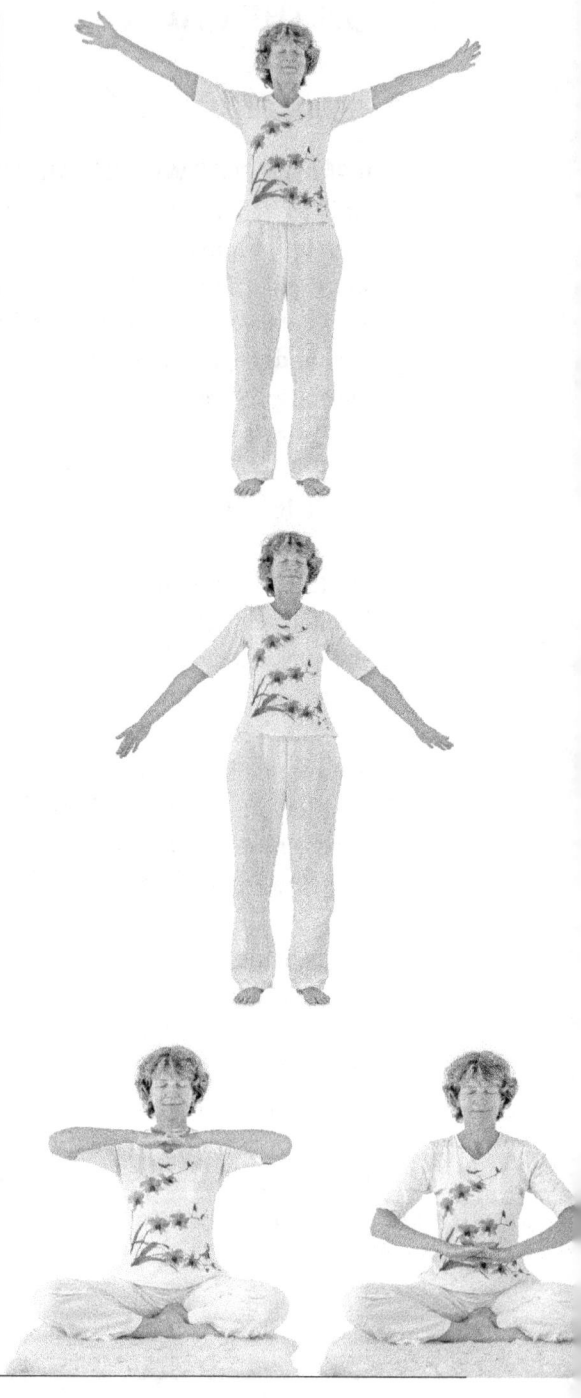

→ continue on next page

3) BACKWARD ARM CIRCLES.

Remain seated with a straight spine. Stretch the arms to the sides and move both arms together in large backward circles. Inhale when the arms come forward and up, and exhale as they go back and down. Continue for **1 minute**.
TO END: Inhale and stretch the arms straight up over your head, exhale, and relax.

4) ARM PUMP VARIATION.

Remain seated with a straight spine. Interlace your fingers with the thumbs touching. Position the hands 4-6 inches (10-15 cm) in front of the chest, both palms facing down. Raise the elbows out to the sides with the forearms parallel to the ground. Inhale and lift the hands to the level of the throat. Exhale and lower them to the level of the navel. Create a steady, pumping motion for **1 minute**. Breathe powerfully.
TO END: Inhale, bring the hands to the level of the heart, suspend the breath briefly, exhale, and relax.

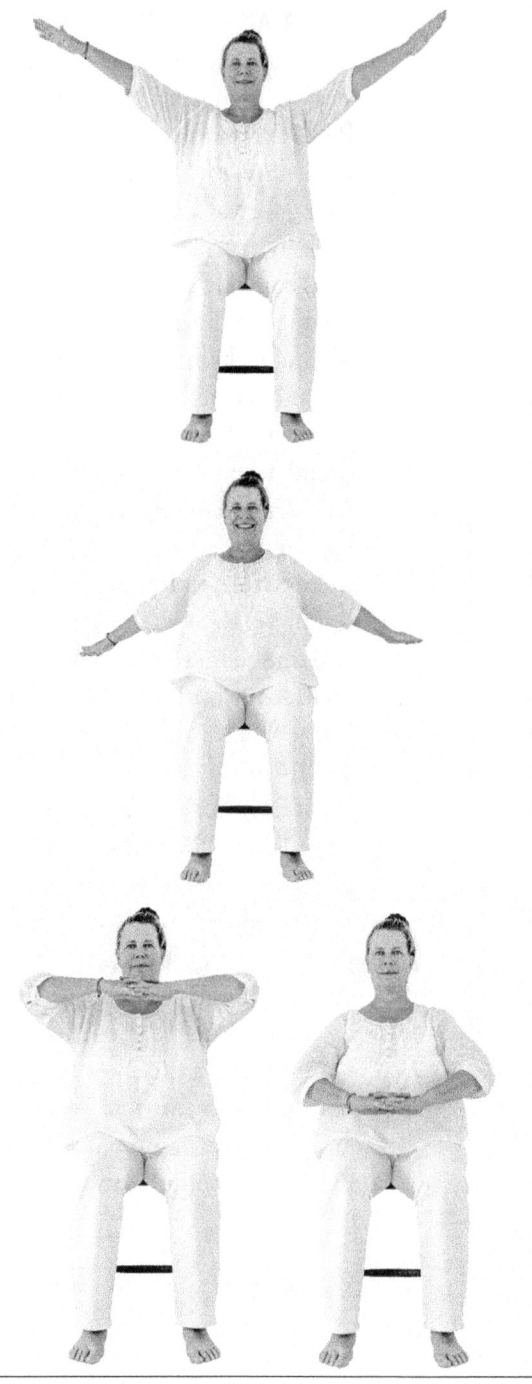

→ continue on next page

5) KIRTAN KRIYA VARIATION.

Stand or remain in Easy Pose with a straight spine and a light Neck Lock. Place the hands beside the shoulders with elbows by your sides and palms facing forward. Close your eyes halfway and fix your gaze downward. Slowly inhale and exhale. The breath is equal on the inhale and the exhale. Mentally chant: **SAA TAA NAA MAA** once on both the inhalation and exhalation. Touch the tip of the thumb to the tip of each finger in the following sequence: thumb tip to the Jupiter (index) finger on **SAA**, thumb tip to Saturn (middle) finger on **TAA**, thumb tip to Sun (ring) finger on **NAA** and thumb tip to Mercury (little) finger on **MAA**. Continue for **3-5 minutes**.

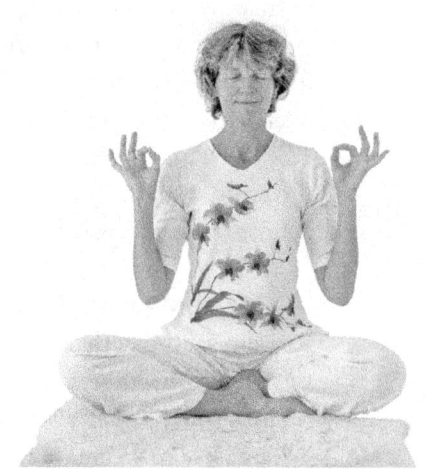

6) PRANAYAM.

Sit in Easy Pose with a straight spine and a light Neck Lock. Gently block the right nostril with the right index finger. Inhale slowly through the left nostril, exhale slowly through rounded lips. The duration of the inhale and exhale is equal, **10 seconds** for each. Continue with this slow breathing pattern for **3 minutes**. Then relax and follow the natural flow of your breath for another **2 minutes**.

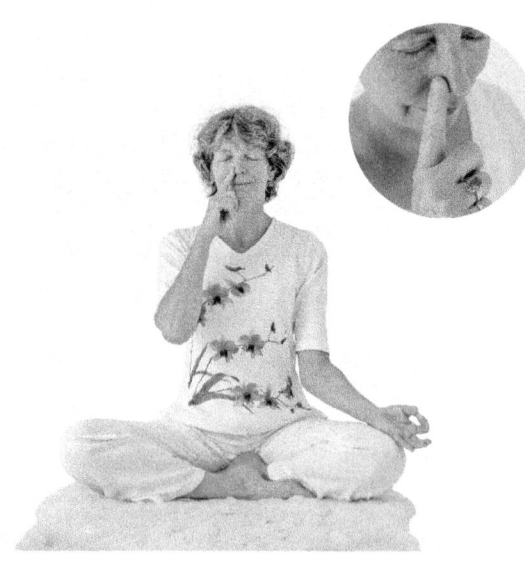

→ continue on next page

5) KIRTAN KRIYA VARIATION.

Remain seated, feet hip-width apart and a straight spine. Place the hands beside the shoulders with the elbows by your sides and the palms facing forward. Close your eyes halfway and gaze downward. Slowly inhale and exhale, the breath equal on the inhale and the exhale. Mentally chant **SAA TAA NAA MAA** once on both the inhalation and exhalation. Touch the tip of the thumb to the tip of each finger in the following sequence: thumb tip to the Jupiter (index) finger on **SAA**, thumb tip to Saturn (middle) finger on **TAA**, thumb tip to Sun (ring) finger on **NAA** and thumb tip to Mercury (little) finger on **MAA**. Continue for **1 minute** to **1 minute and 40 seconds**.

6) PRANAYAM.

Remain seated with a straight spine and the feet hip-width apart. Block the right nostril gently with the right index finger. Inhale slowly through the left nostril, exhale slowly through rounded lips. The duration of inhale and exhale is equal, **10 seconds** for each. Continue this slow breathing pattern for **1 minute**. Then relax and observe the natural flow of your breath for another **1 minute**.

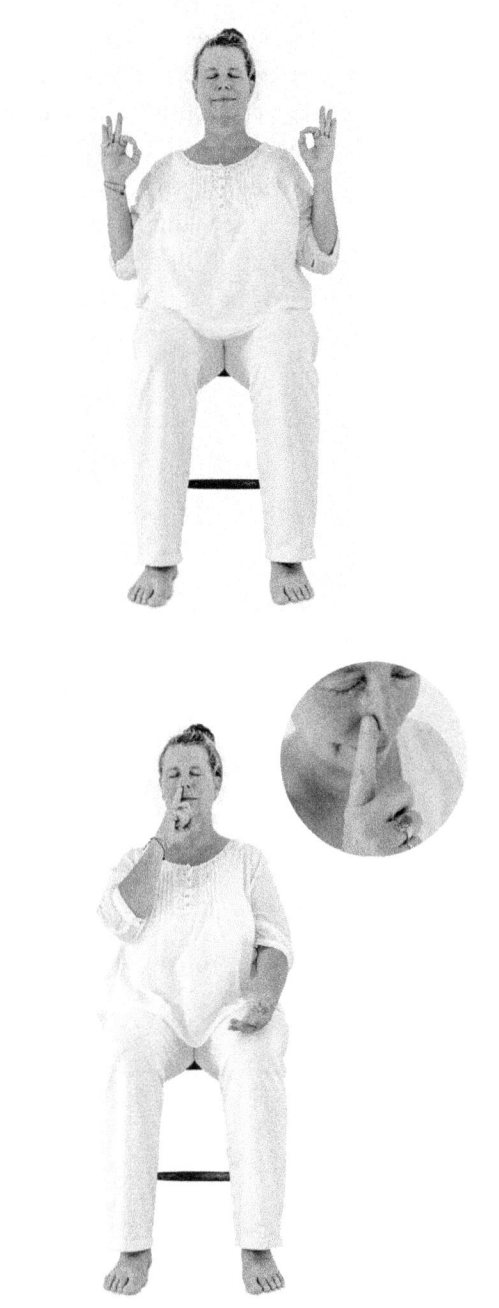

→ continue on next page

Comments: This intermediate level kriya helps you to drop emotional defensiveness and opens up the heart, increasing compassion and sensitivity to others. It calms the mind eliminating unnecessary thoughts and feelings, allowing you to be more present and experience your feelings more clearly.

Comments: This intermediate level kriya helps you to drop emotional defensiveness and opens up the heart, increasing compassion and sensitivity to others. It calms the mind eliminating unnecessary thoughts and feelings, allowing you to be more present and experience your feelings more clearly.

Authors' Recommendation: Deep relaxation. Sit in the back of the chair, so that your lower back is supported. Keep your feet on the ground and connect with the earth. Place your hands open on your upper legs. Relax in this posture for **11 minutes**.

7.3 Meditation for a Calm Heart
September 7, 1981

Sit in Easy Pose with a straight spine and a light Neck Lock.

Mudra: Place the left hand on the Heart Center with fingers pointing to the right, parallel to the ground, thumb relaxed. With the right forearm perpendicular to the ground, raise the right hand as if taking an oath, palm facing forward at the level of the shoulder. Place the right hand in Gyan Mudra, touch the tip of the thumb with the Jupiter (index) finger, and keep the other three fingers extended pointing up.

Eye Focus: Closed or look straight ahead with the eyes 1/10th open.

Breath & Visualization: Concentrate on the flow of the breath. Regulate the breath consciously. Inhale slowly and deeply through both nostrils. Suspend the breath in and raise the chest. Retain it as long as possible. Then exhale smoothly, gradually, and completely. When the breath is totally suspended out, lock the breath out for as long as possible.

Time: Continue for **3-31 minutes**.

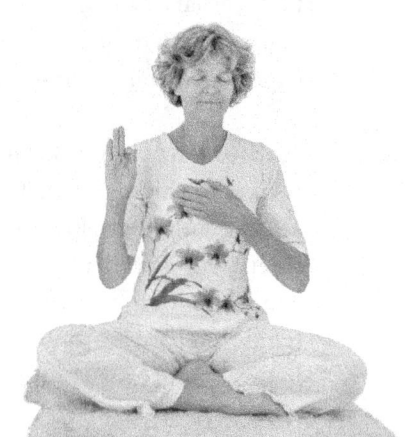

→ continue on next page

ON THE CHAIR

Sit comfortably in a chair with the weight of both feet resting evenly on the ground, with a straight spine, and a light Neck Lock.

Practice as described on the side.

Time: Start with **3 minutes**. If you have more time, try it for three periods of **3 minutes** each, with **1 minute** rest between them, for a total of **11 minutes**.

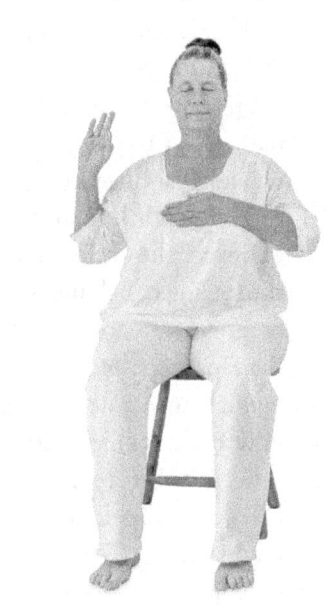

To End: Inhale and exhale strongly. Repeat **2 more times**. Relax.

Comments: The proper home of the subtle force, *praana*, is in the lungs and heart. The left palm is placed at the natural home of *praana*, creating a deep stillness at that point. The right hand that throws you into action and analysis is placed in a receptive, relaxed mudra and put in the position of peace. The entire posture induces the feeling of calmness. It technically creates a still point for the *praana* at the Heart Center. Emotionally, this meditation adds clear perception to your relationships with yourself and others. If you are upset at work or in a personal relationship, sit in this meditation for 3 to 15 minutes before deciding how to act. Then act with your full heart. Physically, this meditation strengthens the lungs and heart. This meditation is perfect for beginners. It broadens awareness of the breath, and it conditions the lungs. When you hold the breath in or out for "as long as possible," you should not gasp or be under strain when you let the breath move again. For an advanced practice of concentration and rejuvenation, build the meditation up to 31 minutes.

CHAPTER 8
Self Expression

—

When you speak on the human level, when you speak about a purpose or a mission which is beyond you, then you try to reach the hearts of other people. Your language changes, your word changes, your sound changes.
— YOGI BHAJAN, MARCH 20, 1995

This chapter will focus on the fifth chakra or the Vishudda, the throat center. The chakra relates to the theme of truth and expression, as well as how to remove blocks to self-expression. You will become aware of this theme and learn what you can do to achieve balance. The fifth chakra is located near the neck and voice box. It is associated with the ability to communicate, the truth, knowing, and self-expression. This chakra is connected with teaching and being a teacher, and the creative power of the word.

Which aspect of this chakra do you most relate to, and which one do you relate to the least? For example maybe you relate to the concept of truth and this makes you feel balanced, but you sometimes have difficulty in communicating clearly and so that makes you feel unbalanced. This can give you an idea of which aspects to focus on in your own development.

The fifth chakras' motto is: *I communicate openly.* Blue is the color associated with this chakra. The element is ether. The subtle perception is sound. The organs associated with this chakra are the trachea (or windpipe), neck, cervical vertebrae, and thyroid.

Chakra imbalances manifest as denial, poor expressive abilities, not expressing one's opinion, insecurity, shyness and lethargy. In the physical body, a weak fifth chakra can manifest with problems with the voice, throat, neck problems, as well as thyroid issues. With a poorly developed fifth chakra you may find yourself feeling unable to express who you are and even have stage fright, or have continuing difficult and frustrating communication patterns.

As adults, we get to know our own truth. The throat chakra is associated with communication and expression, as well as listening. At this point you can simultaneously understand what the other person is saying, and at the same time be aware of your own truth. Transformation, the ability to enter new spheres of influence, and spiritual freedom are all aspects of this chakra in balance.

What affects the fifth chakra: Exercises that focus on the throat, nose, and ears. Exercises that focus on neck alignment and increasing mobility of the neck and cervical spine. Listening to music, singing mantras, conversing, writing letters, journaling, and learning a new language are all examples of expressive activities. This chakra can be experienced through listening and sound, for example, by listening to music and by singing.

The first kriya, the *Kriya to Develop Command Reflex and Alertness*, improves your responsiveness and how you respond in unexpected situations. This kriya works on connecting the hemispheres of the brain and the ability to focus your thoughts before you act. The second *Kriya for Intuition and Communication* builds on the subtlety of intuition and enhances the ability to communicate. The meditation *Aad Naad Kriya* enhances your speech and helps you be heard. The *Aad Naad* meditation also helps with communication, reducing anxiety, and improving clarity and harmony in a relationship.

Finally, the additional resource *Universal Rules of Communication* gives you guidelines for understanding how to create better communication. These rules for communication have at their center the idea that we communicate not just for the sake of our own feelings, but we communicate to create a better and more harmonious future. A strong fifth chakra is about expression that can generate truth, harmony, and balanced relationships.

8.1 Kriya to Develop Command Reflex and Alertness
June 27, 1984

Practice the kriya 2 times in one sitting.

1) CLAPPING WITH CHANTING.
Sit in Easy Pose with a straight spine and a light Neck Lock. Move and chant in the following sequence: extend the arms straight forward at the level of the heart and clap on **SAA**; open the arms straight out to the sides with palms facing up on **TAA**; keep the arms out to the sides and turn the palms facing down on **NAA**; raise the arms straight up and clap on **MAA**. Continue for **1 minute**.

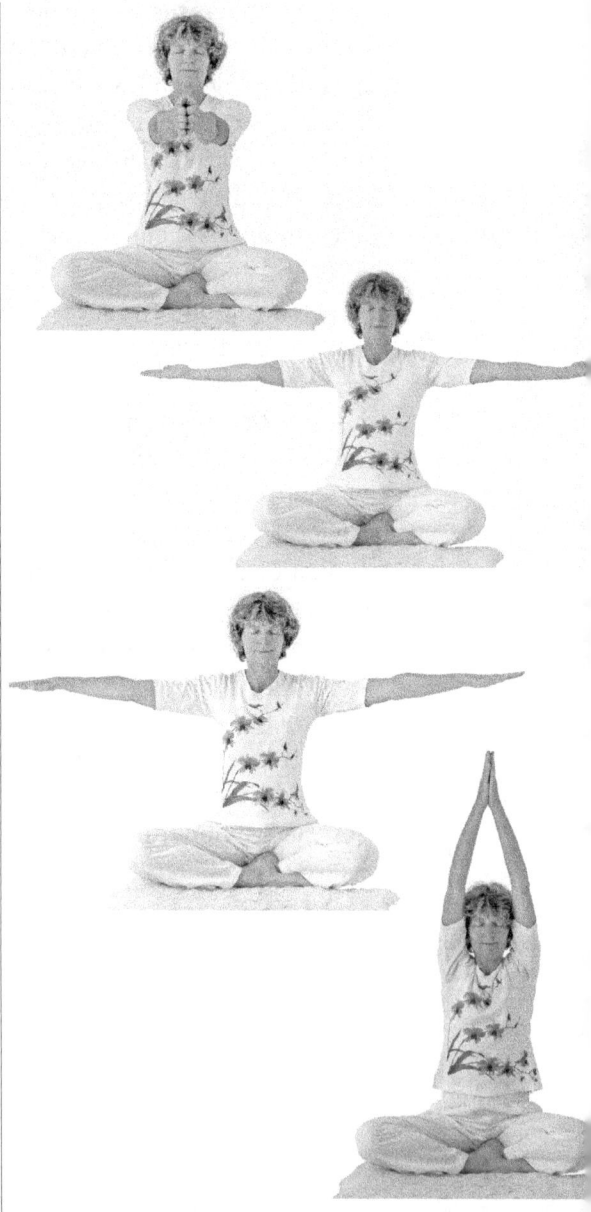

→ continue on next page

ON THE CHAIR

Practice the kriya 2 times in one sitting.

1) CLAPPING WITH CHANTING.
Sit in a chair, feet hip-width apart and even weight on both feet with a straight spine and a light Neck Lock. Move and chant in the following sequence: extend the arms straight forward at the level of the heart and clap on **SAA**; open the arms straight out to the sides with palms facing up on **TAA**; keep the arms out to the sides and turn the palms facing down on **NAA**; raise the arms straight up and clap on **MAA**. Continue for **1 minute**.

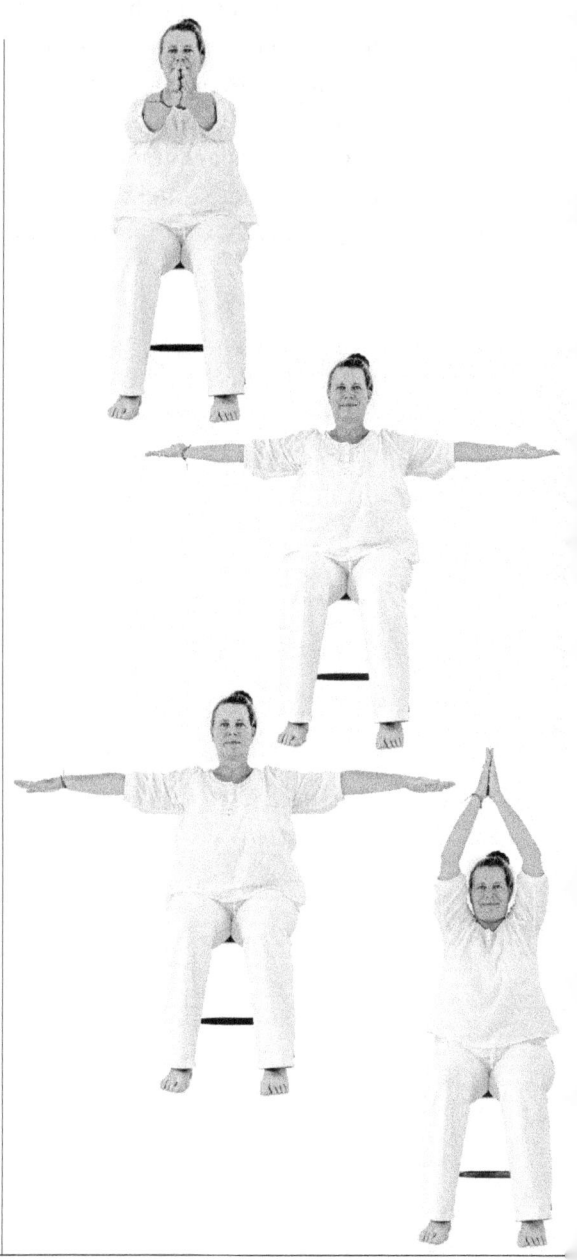

→ continue on next page

2) REVERSE CLAPPING WITH CHANTING. Remain in Easy Pose and reverse the sequence of exercise 1 as follows: Raise the arms straight up and clap on **SAA**; extend the arms straight out to the sides with palms facing down on **TAA**; keep the arms out to the sides and turn the palms facing up on **NAA**; bring the arms straight forward and clap on **MAA**. Continue for **2 minutes**.

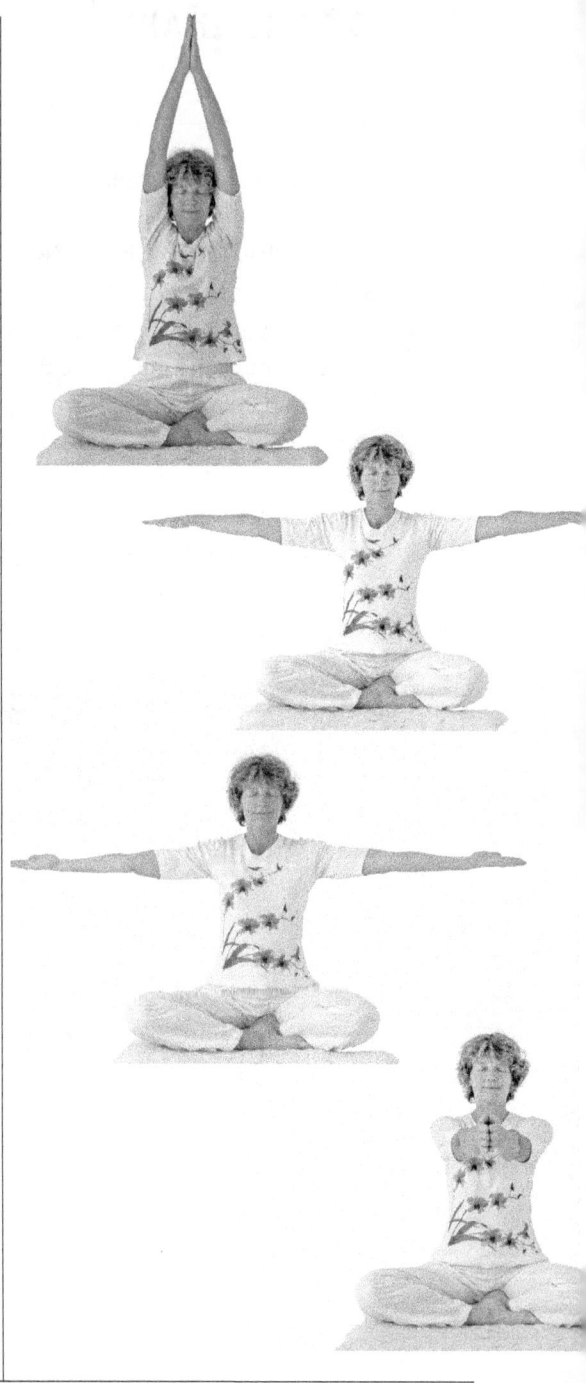

→ continue on next page

2) REVERSE CLAPPING WITH CHANTING.
Remain seated and reverse the sequence of exercise 1 as follows: Raise the arms straight up and clap on **SAA**; extend the arms straight out to the sides with palms facing down on **TAA**; keep the arms out to the sides and turn the palms facing up on **NAA**; bring the arms straight forward and clap on **MAA**. Continue for **1 minute**.

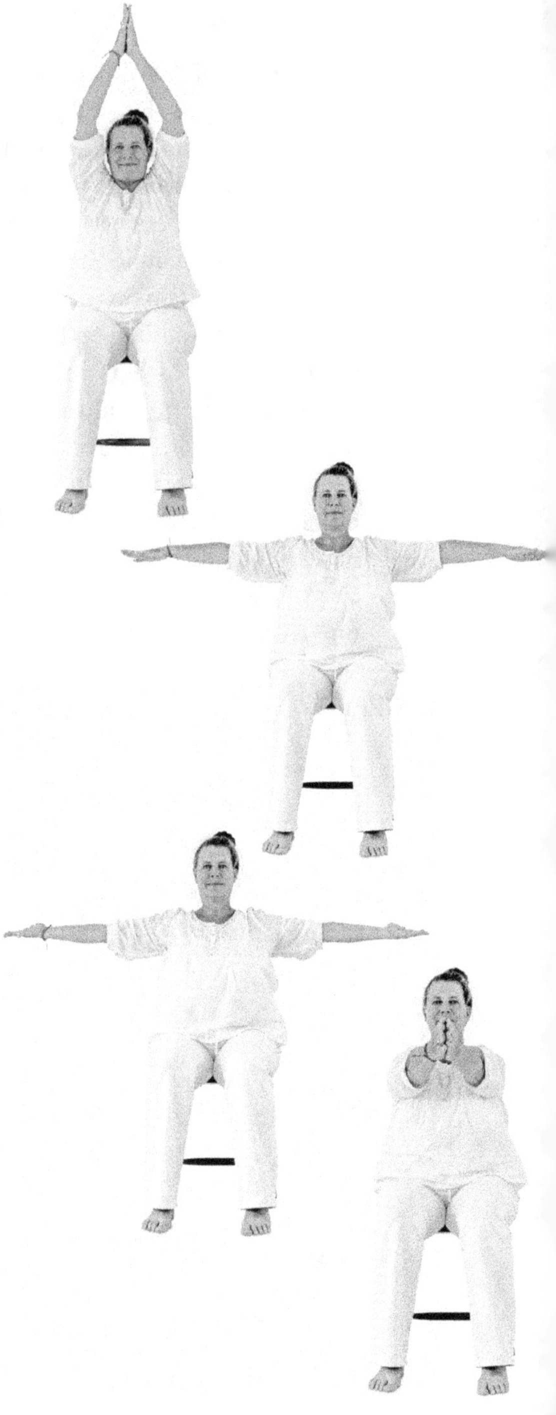

→ continue on next page

3) YOGA MUDRA VARIATION.
Sit on the heels in Rock Pose with a straight spine and a light Neck Lock. Place the hands behind the back and interlock the fingers with palms facing up. Move and chant in the following sequence: stand up on the knees on **SAA**; remain standing on the knees and bend from the hips, place the forehead on the ground and raise the arms behind your back as far as possible on **TAA**; rise up standing on the knees, hands relaxed at the base of the spine on **NAA**; sit in Rock Pose, hands at the base of the spine on **MAA**. Continue for **2 minutes**.

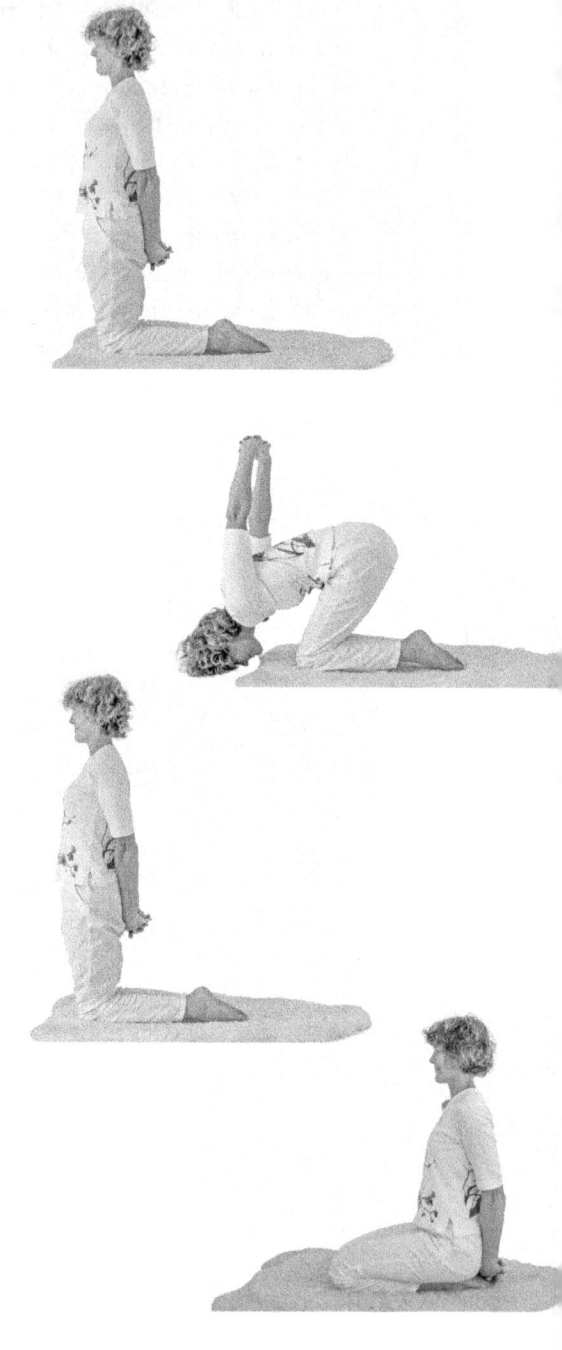

→ continue on next page

3) YOGA MUDRA VARIATION.

Sit at the front of the chair, the feet hip-width apart, a bit further away from you. Place the hands behind the back and interlock the fingers with palms facing up. Use a scarf if necessary or hold the back of the chair throughout the exercise. Move and chant in the following sequence: remain seated with a straight spine slide your left foot under the chair on **SAA**; bend the upper body forward, raise the arms behind your back as high if possible on **TAA**; rise up to the starting position, hands relaxed at the base of the spine on **NAA**; bring the left foot back on the ground, hands at the base of the spine. Continue for **30 seconds**. Repeat the exercise with the right foot under the chair for **30 seconds**.

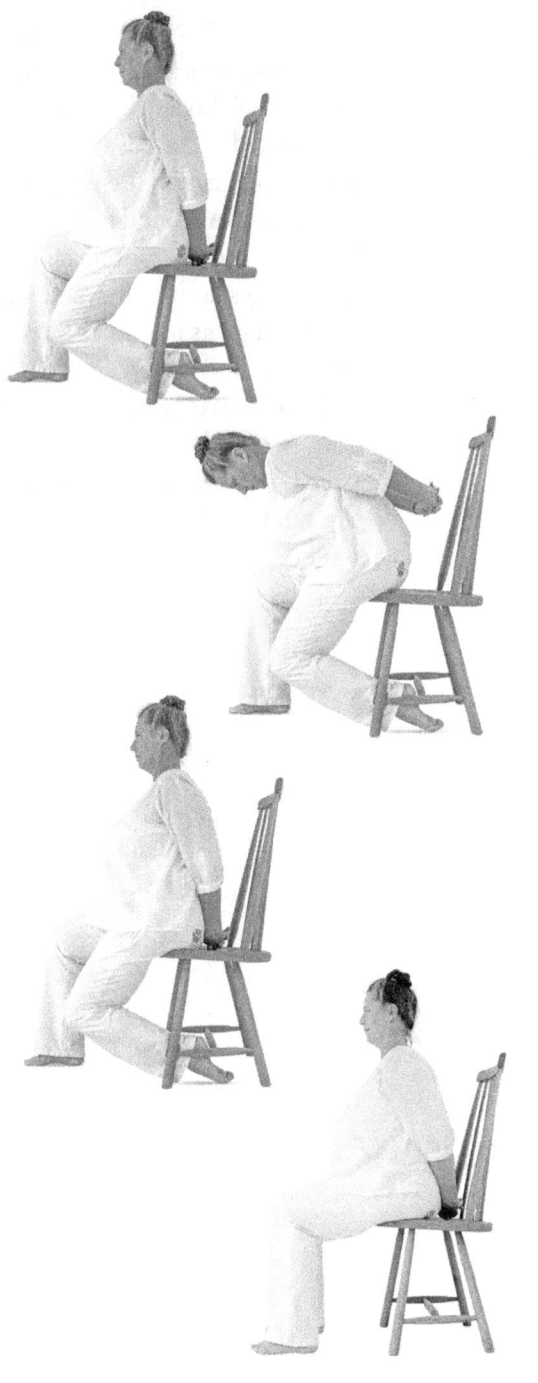

→ continue on next page

4) MIRACLE BEND VARIATION.
Stand up with a straight spine and a light Neck Lock. The hands are interlocked at the base of the spine. Move and chant in the following sequence: **SAA** bend forward from the hips bringing your forehead as close to your legs as possible, and raise the arms as high as possible; **TAA** stand up with arms relaxed down; **NAA** arch backwards as far as you can, arms relaxed behind you; **MAA** stand back up with hands at the base of the spine. Continue for **2 minutes**.

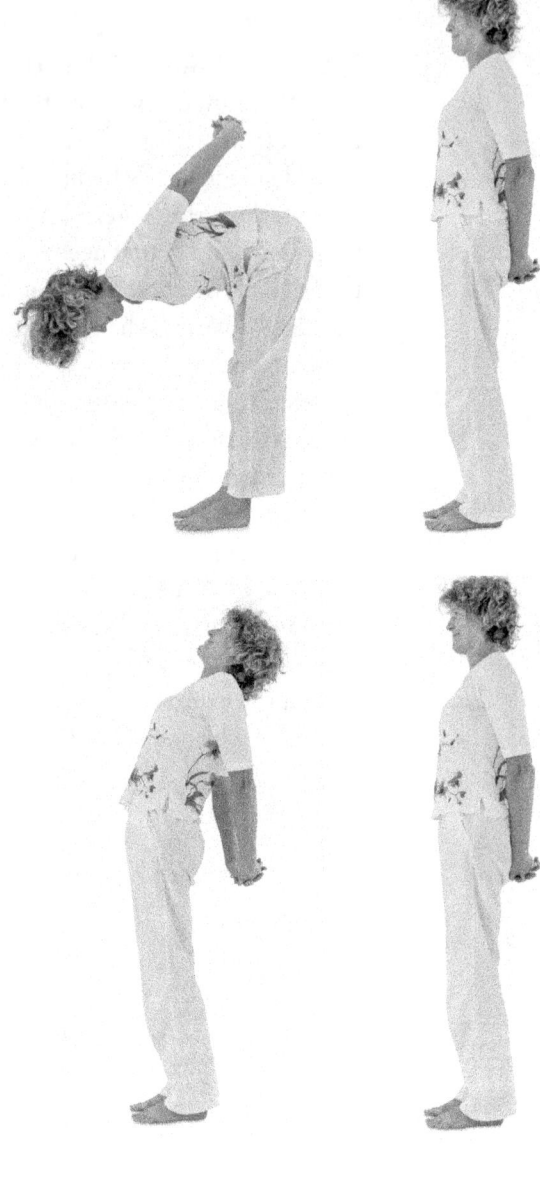

→ continue on next page

4) MIRACLE BEND VARIATION.

Remain seated at the front of the chair with the fingers interlocked behind the back. Use a scarf if necessary, or hold the back of the seat throughout the exercise. Move and chant in the following sequence: **SAA** bend forward from the hips bringing your forehead as close to your legs as possible and raise the arms as high as possible; **TAA** rise up with arms relaxed down; **NAA** pull Root Lock, open your chest and arch backwards as far as you can, arms relaxed behind you; **MAA** come back seated with a straight spine and the hands at the base of the spine. Continue for **1 minute**.

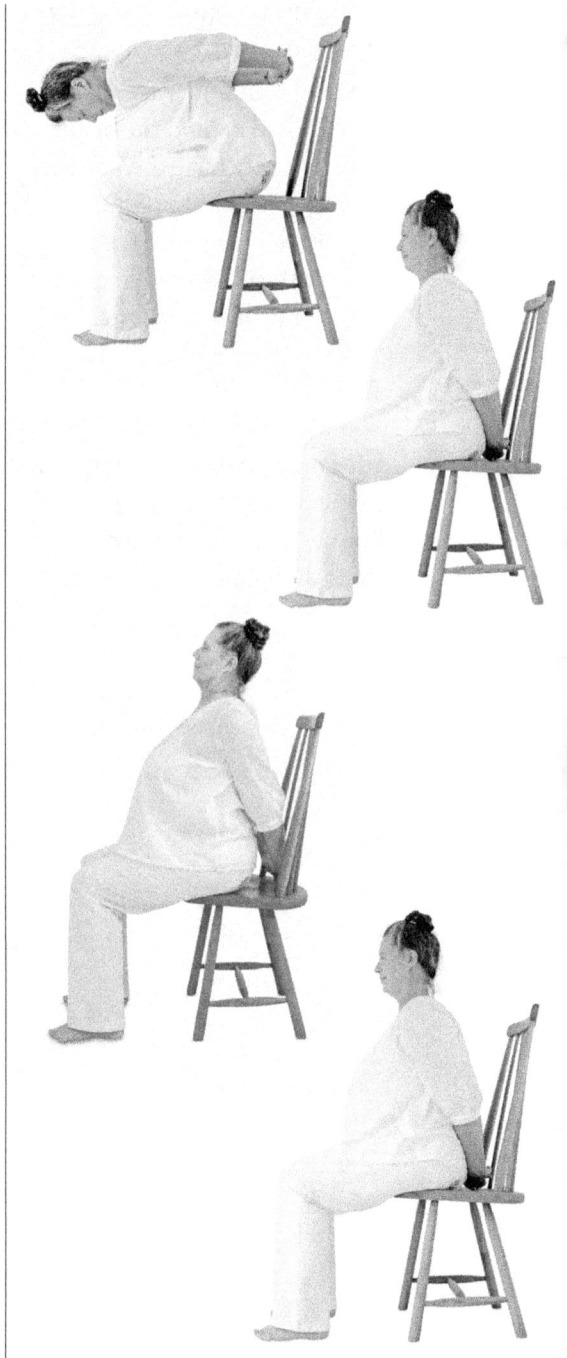

→ continue on next page

5) STANDING KNEE RAISES WITH YOGA MUDRA.

Remain standing with fingers interlocked behind the back. Alternatively raise the knees as high as possible. Simultaneously with each knee, raise the arms up behind the back as high as possible. Continue for **4 minutes**.

Comments: The movements with sounds in these exercises build the connection between the two hemispheres of the brain. This connection allows you to focus your thoughts before you act.

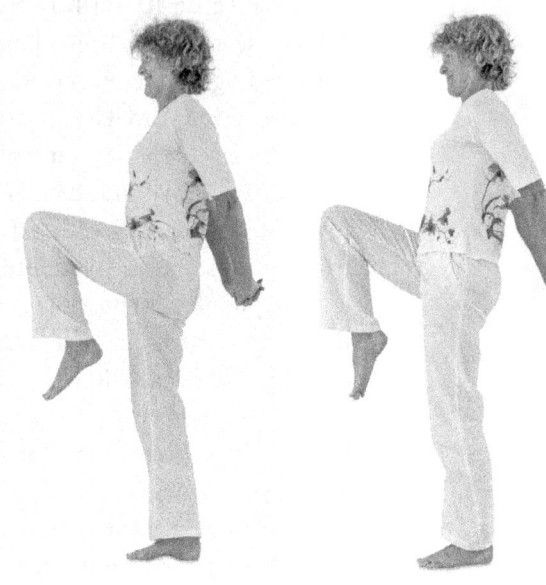

5) KNEE RAISES WITH YOGA MUDRA. Remain seated at the front of the chair. Interlock the fingers behind the back. Use a scarf if necessary, or hold the back of the seat throughout the exercise. Alternatively, raise the knees as high as possible. Simultaneously with each knee, raise the arms up behind the back as high as possible. Continue for **2 minutes**.

Authors' Recommendation: Deep relaxation. Sit in the back of the chair, relax completely for **10 minutes**.

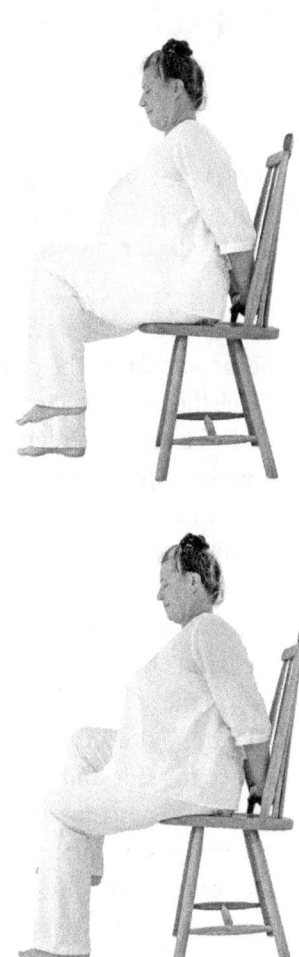

8.2 Kriya for Intuition and Communication
Summer 1983

1) ARM MOVEMENTS IN CROW POSE. Stand with the feet hip-width apart and a light Neck Lock. Squat down into a Crow Pose, keep the knees, ankles and feet in parallel alignment, and the spine as perpendicular to the ground as possible. Place the hands facing each other in front of the Heart Center with approximately 6 inches (15 cm) between them. The elbows are out to the sides and forearms parallel to the ground. With an 8 count rhythm (approximately 1 count per second), move in the following sequence:
a) Extend the right arm straight out to the side and back.
b) Extend the left arm straight out to the side and back.
c) Extend both arms straight up as you stand up.
d) Return to the original position in Crow Pose.
e) Extend the right arm straight out to the side and back.
f) Extend the left arm straight out to the side and back.
g) Extend both arms straight out to the sides.
h) Return to the original position.
Continue for **1 minute** counting with the movement. Then begin chanting **SAA TAA NAA MAA SAA TAA NAA MAA** in rhythm and continue for **1-2 minutes** more.

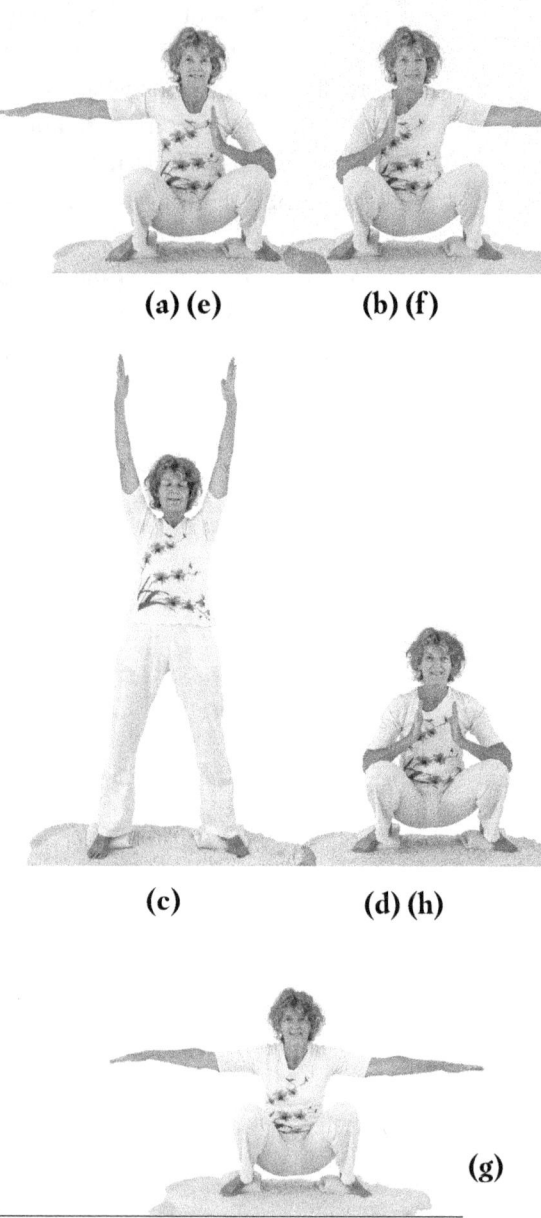

(a) (e)   (b) (f)

(c)   (d) (h)

(g)

→ continue on next page

ON THE CHAIR

1) ARM MOVEMENTS.
Sit in a chair, feet hip-width apart and even weight on both feet with a straight spine, and a light Neck Lock. Place the hands facing each other in front of the Heart Center with approximately 6 inches (15 cm) between them. The elbows are out to the sides and forearms parallel to the ground. With an 8 count rhythm (approximately 1 count per second), move in the following sequence:
a) Extend the right arm straight out to the side and back.
b) Extend the left arm straight out to the side and back.
c) Extend both arms straight up.
d) Return to the original position.
e) Extend the right arm straight out to the side and back.
f) Extend the left arm straight out to the side and back.
g) Extend both arms straight out to the sides.
h) Return to the original position. Continue for **1 minute** counting with the movement. Then begin chanting **SAA TAA NAA MAA SAA TAA NAA MAA** in rhythm and continue for **1 more minute**.

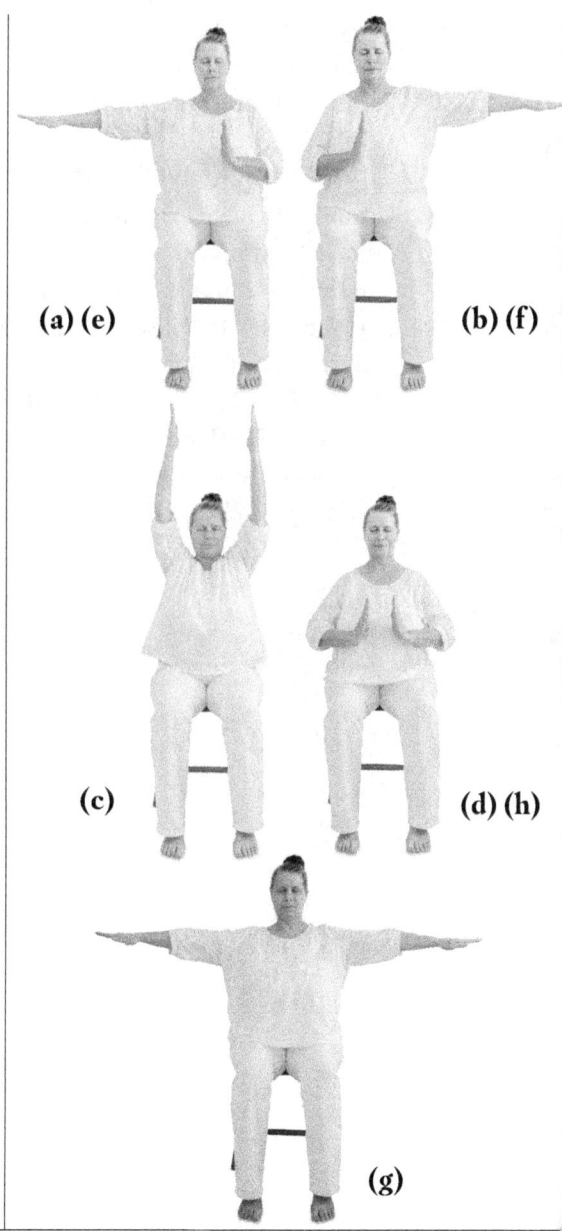

→ continue on next page

2) STANDING TORSO CIRCLES.
Stand up, feet a little wider than shoulder-width apart, hands on the hips with a straight spine, and a light Neck Lock. Rotate the torso in large circles from the hips. Continue for **2 minutes**.

3) YOGIC KICKS WITH CHANTING.
Stand with feet closer together on the balls of the feet with the hands on the hips. Shift the weight to one foot and kick the other foot forward, alternately, at a quick pace. Chant loudly, **HUM DUM HAR HAR, HAR HAR HUM DUM**[1]. Continue rhythmically for **3 minutes**. Continue the Yogic Kicks and chant Jaap Sahib, if available, for as long as you want.

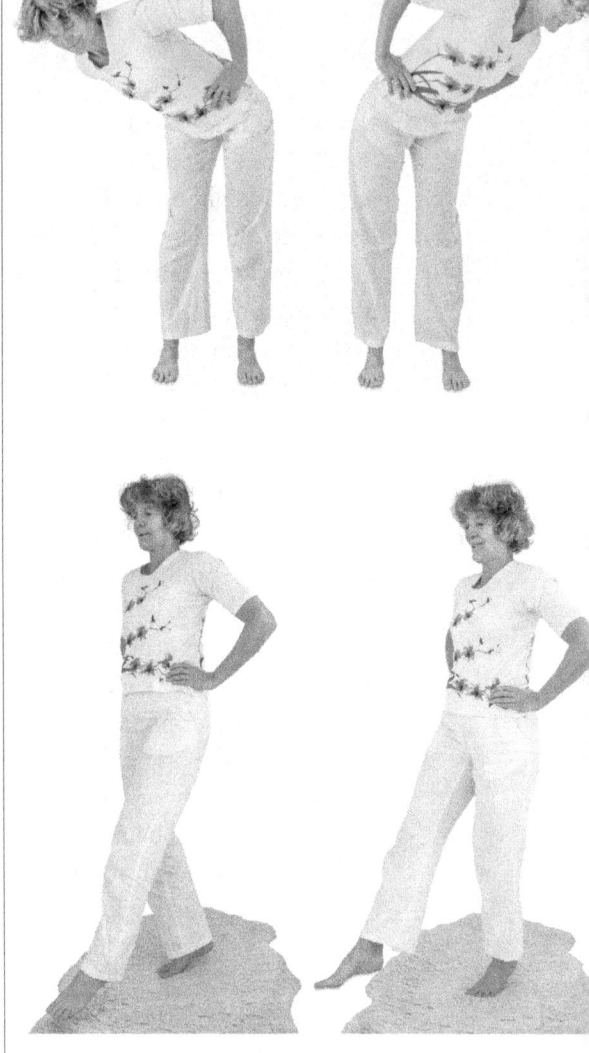

---

1 Authors' Note: The mantra Hum Dum Har Har, Har Har Hum Dum opens up the heart chakra.

2) STANDING TORSO CIRCLES.
Remain seated with your feet hip-width apart and the hands on the hips. Rotate the torso from the hips in large circles. Continue for **1 minute**.

3) YOGIC KICKS WITH CHANTING.
Remain seated with your feet hip-width apart and the hands on the hips. Come onto the ball of the feet and, alternatively kick the feet forward. Chant loudly, **HUM DUM HAR HAR, HAR HAR HUM DUM**[1] rhythmically for **1 minute**. Continue the Yogic Kicks and chant Jaap Sahib, if available, for as long as you want.

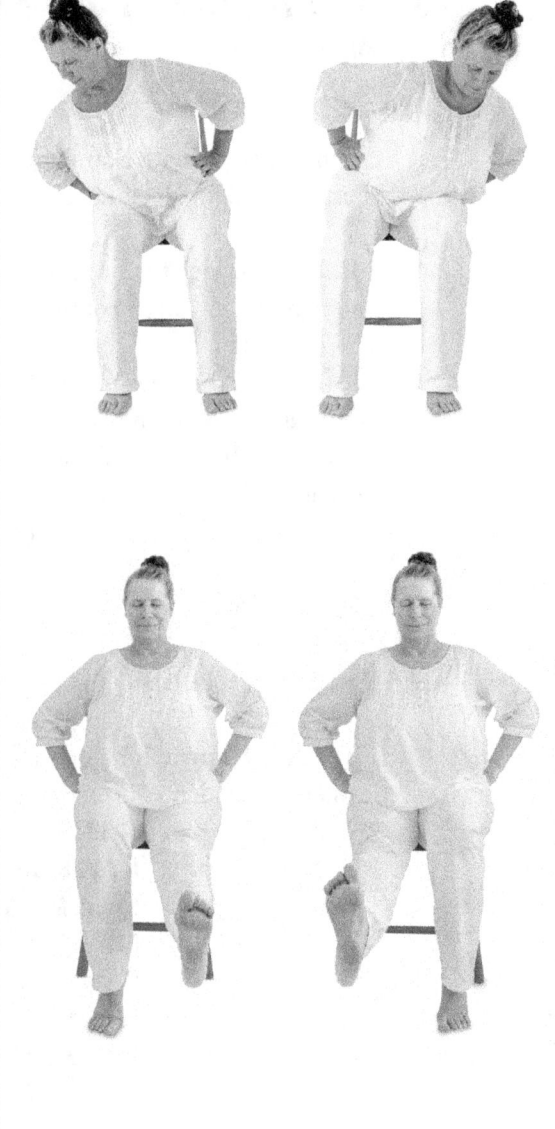

---

[1] Authors' Note: The mantra Hum Dum Har Har, Har Har Hum Dum opens up the heart chakra.

8.3 Meditation: Aad Naad Kriya
April 23, 1978

Sit in Easy Pose with a straight spine and a light Neck Lock.

Mudra: Interlock the fingers with the right fingers on top of the corresponding left fingers. The palms are together, the sides of the thumbs touch and are stretched back so that they point straight up. The arms are relaxed at the sides with the hands held in front of the body between the solar plexus and the Heart Center. Keep the thumbs stretched up.

Eye Focus: Closed.

Breath & Mantra: Inhale deeply, exhale as the mantra is chanted once.

> RAA RAA
> RAA RAA
> MAA MAA
> MAA MAA
> SAA SAA
> SAA SAT
> HAREE HAR
> HAREE HAR

Time: Continue for **11 minutes**. You can extend the time to **31** or **62 minutes** or longer.

To End: Inhale deeply, suspend the breath for at least **15 seconds**, exhale through the mouth. Repeat **2 more times**.

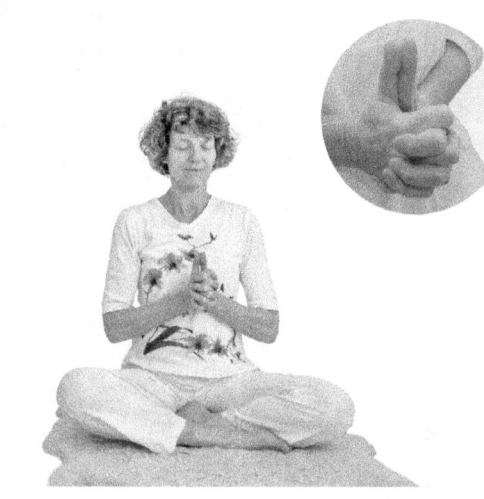

→ continue on next page

ON THE CHAIR

Sit comfortably in a chair with the weight of both feet resting evenly on the ground, with a straight spine, and a light Neck Lock.

Practice as described on the side.

Time: Start with **3 minutes** and gradually build up the time.

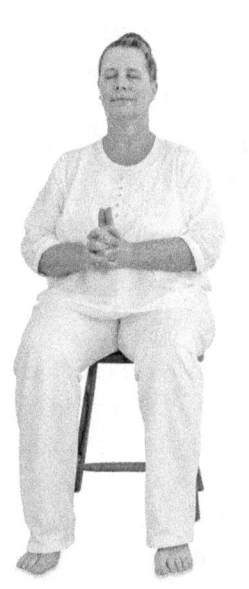
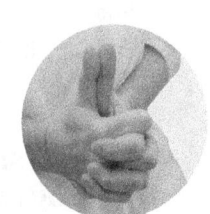

Additional Exercise:
Universal rules of communication

Originally published in The Aquarian Teacher Conscious Communication

Share your impressions on intuitive speaking with one another and use the Universal rules for Communication to do so.

Universal rules of communication, by Yogi Bhajan

Rule One: You are communicating for a better tomorrow, not to spoil today.
Rule Two: Whatever you are going to say is going to live forever. And you have to live through it. Therefore take care you don't have to live through the mud of your own communication.
Rule Three: One wrong word said can do much more wrong than you can imagine or even estimate.
Rule Four: Words spoken are a chance for communication. Don't turn them into a war.
Rule Five: When you communicate once, you have to communicate again. Don't make the road rough.

CHAPTER 9
Purpose

—

Meditation is nothing but taking a mental shower, cleaning yourself and answering the call of nature, that's the mantra.

— YOGI BHAJAN, SEPTEMBER 12, 1989

In this chapter, you will practice concentration, developing your intuition, allowing the mastery of your human spirit, and knowing clearly what is good for you. You will become aware of these themes and learn what you can do to achieve balance. The focus of this chapter is the sixth chakra or the Ajna. The brow chakra, or Third Eye Point, is located between the eyebrows in the middle of the forehead. This chakra governs concentration and determination, intuition, sharp perception, projection, as well as promoting purposefulness. The strengths of the sixth chakra include intuition, enhanced wisdom, and even the subtle development of these qualities, such as clairvoyance. The sixth chakra is also the gateway to the upper chakras, where we move beyond the elements of the material world and into the subtle energies represented by meditation.

The sixth chakras' motto is: *I see things through my intuition.* Indigo is the color associated with this chakra. The organs are the brain, eyes, ears, nose, nasal cavity, and pituitary gland.

Chakra imbalances can manifest as confusion, depression, thinking too schematically, rationalizing everything or over-intellectualizing, and little spiritual development. A weak sixth chakra can feel like not knowing your purpose, feeling directionless and locked in the process of the mind.

The sixth chakra is where we begin to develop the capacity to meditate. During yoga practice, we focus on the Third Eye Point to strengthen concentration and avoid distractions, which are also qualities of the sixth chakra. With this focus, thoughts are allowed to settle and pass; then you will learn to master your mind. More awareness emerges, as well as improved intuition and spiritual development. You have more time and attention to devote to spiritual development as you get older, and the sixth chakra naturally strengthens.

What has an impact on your sixth chakra: Kriyas and meditations that affect the pituitary gland, intuition, or strengthening your Third Eye Point; all kriyas with bowing or resting your forehead on the ground.

The sixth chakra is enhanced by singing mantras, which help you allow your thoughts to pass. New experiences with like-minded people also impact this chakra.

The first exercise's breathing practice called *Becoming Aware of Your Breath* makes you aware of your breath and brings you into the present moment. The *Kriya to Become Intuitive* strengthens your intuition. These exercises gently work on the pituitary gland, a master gland in the brain. They recharge and enrich your energy and counteract frustration and depression.

Following that, the *Meditation for Powerful Energy* helps you clear your mind and balance your brain, so that insight can emerge. In this meditation, you chant "Ong" which vibrates through the skull when chanting it. It is the sound of the sixth chakra, the center of consciousness, and by singing it you can experience your joy and connection with your own being.

9.1 Becoming Aware of Your Breath
Originally published in Praana, Pranee, Pranayam

To get the full benefits from praanayam, it is essential that we meditate on our breathing as we practice. We may keep other things in our awareness as well, but we always keep track of what our breath is doing. Here are a few ways to keep your attention on the breath:

Sit in Easy Pose with a straight spine and a light Neck Lock.
1) Listen to the sounds of your breath, pay attention to tone, rhythm, speed and tension (difficult or fluid).
2) Visualize how the breath enters the body, fills up the lungs and then leaves the body again, emptying your lungs.
3) Visualize how the diaphragm is pulled downward on the inhalation and comes back up again on the exhalation.
4) Feel how your chest expands while inhaling and contracts again while exhaling.
5) Feel the breath as it enters through the nose while breathing in, and contracts again while breathing out.
6) Feel the temperature in your nose: it is colder on the inhalation and warmer on the exhalation. Imagine the breath in every cell of your body. Feel the breath, become one with your breath.

Comments: While breathing in, the sides expand, the diaphragm flattens, and more space for the lungs is created. At the exhalation, the sides flatten and the diaphragm expands, causing the lungs to have less space and empty themselves.

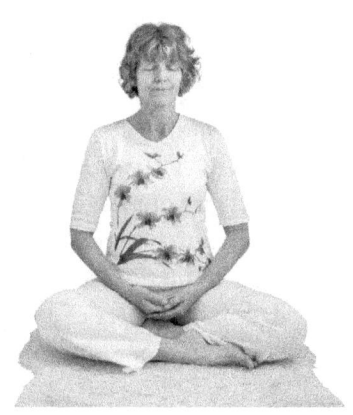

ON THE CHAIR

Sit comfortably in a chair with the weight of both feet resting evenly on the ground, with a straight spine, and a light Neck Lock.

Practice as described on the side.

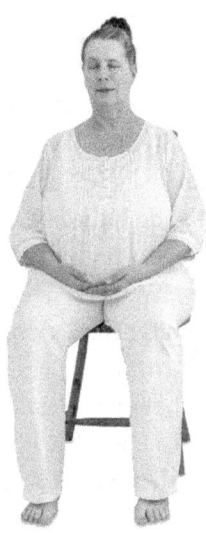

9.2 Kriya to Become Intuitive
March 9, 1998

There are no breaks between the exercises.

1) RIGHT HAND JUPITER.
Sit in Easy Pose with a straight spine and a light Neck Lock. Place the left hand on the Heart Center with the fingers pointing to the right, thumb relaxed. Make fist with the right hand, Jupiter (index) finger extended and the other fingers held down with the thumb. Bring the right elbow to the side of the body, bend the elbow, with the forearm perpendicular to the ground, palm facing forward and the Jupiter finger pointing straight up. Consciously keep your back very straight. Elongate your back and put as little weight on your buttocks as possible. Close the eyes and inhale slowly and deeply through the nose, suspend the breath, and then exhale slowly with a whistle through the mouth. Continue for **7 minutes**.
Imagine that something very pure and divine in you is calling. Reach out and make contact with your own Infinity. Create a feeling of being exalted by your own self.

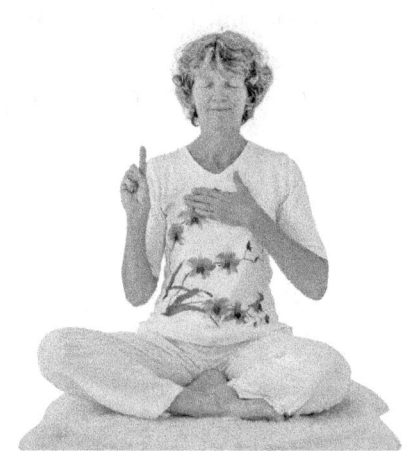

→ continue on next page

ON THE CHAIR

1) RIGHT HAND JUPITER.
Sit in a chair, feet hip-width apart and even weight on both feet with a straight spine and a light Neck Lock. Place your left hand on the Heart Center with the fingers pointing to the right, thumb relaxed. Make fist with the right hand, Jupiter (index) finger extended and the other fingers held down with the thumb. Bring the right elbow to the side of the body, bend the elbow, with the forearm perpendicular to the ground, palm facing forward and the Jupiter finger pointing straight up. Consciously keep your back very straight. Elongate your back and put as little weight on your buttocks as possible. Close the eyes and inhale slowly and deeply through the nose, suspend the breath, and then exhale slowly with a whistle through the mouth. Continue for **2 minutes and 20 seconds**.
Imagine that something very pure and divine in you is calling. Reach out and make contact with your own Infinity. Create a feeling of being exalted by your own self.

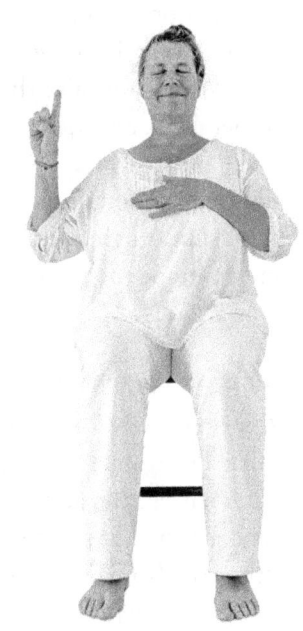

→ continue on next page

2) LEFT HAND JUPITER.

Remain in Easy Pose. Place the right hand on top of your head or slightly above with the fingers pointing to the left. Make fist with the left hand, Jupiter (index) finger extended and the other fingers held down with the thumb. Bring the left elbow to the side of the body, raise the forearm perpendicular to the ground, palm facing forward and the Jupiter finger pointing straight up. Keep the spine pulled up straight. Close your eyes and continue the breath sequence from Exercise 1 for **4 minutes**.

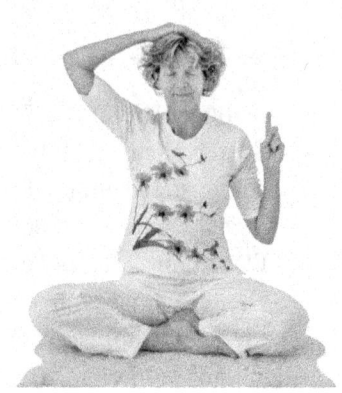

3) PRAYER POSE VARIATION.

Remain in Easy Pose and press the palms flat against each other in Prayer Mudra. Raise the arms up over the head. Keep your spine straight and stretch up from the armpits. Continue with the same breath for **2 ½ minutes**. *In this exercise, you consciously recirculate your energy to give your body new life.*

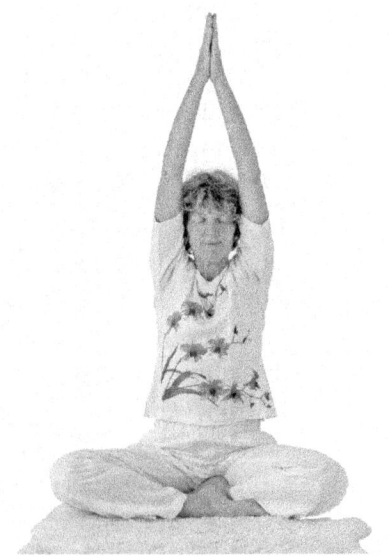

→ continue on next page

2) LEFT HAND JUPITER.

Remain seated with the feet hip-width apart. Place the right hand on top of your head or slightly above with the fingers pointing to the left. Make fist with the left hand, Jupiter (index) finger extended and the other fingers held down with the thumb. Bring the left elbow to the side of the body, raise the forearm perpendicular to the ground, palm facing forward, and the Jupiter finger pointing straight up. Keep the spine pulled up straight. Close your eyes and continue the breath sequence from Exercise 1 for **1 minute and 20 seconds**.

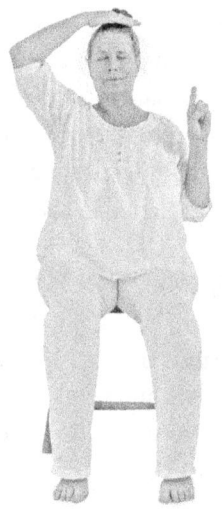

3) PRAYER POSE VARIATION.

Remain seated and press the palms flat against each other in Prayer Mudra. Raise the arms up over the head. Keep your spine straight and stretch up from the armpits. Continue with the same breath for **1 minute**. *In this exercise, you consciously recirculate your energy to give your body new life.*

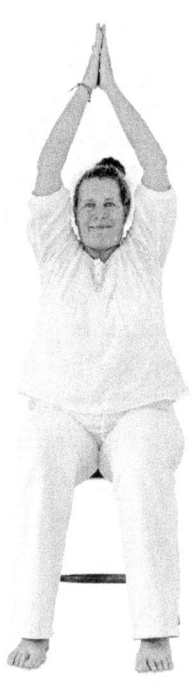

→ continue on next page

4) MEDITATE.

Remain in Easy Pose. Place the left hand on the Heart Center and place the right hand on top of the left. Relax and listen to the music for **3 ½ minutes**. ("Rakhe Rakhanhar" by Singh Kaur was played in the original class.)

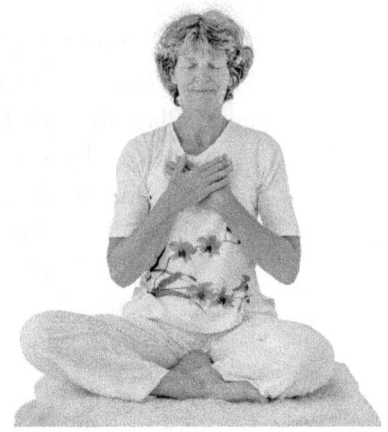

5) NAVEL PRESS WITH CHANTING.

Remain in Easy Pose and place both hands on the Navel Point. Chant **HAR** and firmly press the navel with each repetition of **HAR**. Chant with the eyes closed for **3 minutes**.

TO END: Lock the arms in front of the body, with each hand grasping the opposite elbow. The forearms are parallel to the ground at shoulder height. Inhale, suspend the breath for **5-10 seconds**, squeeze the spine, and tighten all the muscles of the body. Exhale. Repeat this sequence **2 more times**.

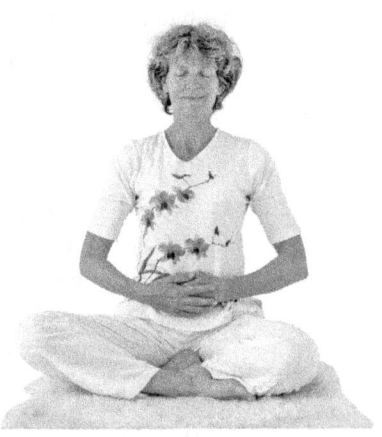

Comments: This kriya gently works on the pituitary recharging your energy and reducing frustration and depression.

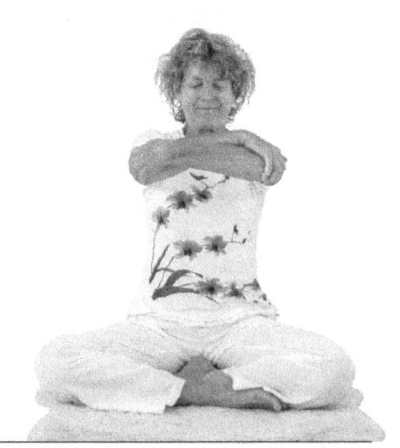

4) MEDITATE.
Remain seated with the feet hip-width apart. Place the left hand on the Heart Center and place the right hand on top of the left. Relax and listen to the music for **1 minute and 10 seconds**. ("Rakhe Rakhanhar" by Singh Kaur was played in the original class.)

5) NAVEL PRESS WITH CHANTING.
Remain seated and place both hands on the Navel Point. Chant **HAR** and firmly press the navel with each repetition of **HAR.** Chant with the eyes closed for **1 minute**.
TO END: Lock the arms in front of the body, with each hand grasping the opposite elbow. The forearms are parallel to the ground at shoulder height. Inhale, suspend the breath briefly, squeeze the spine and tighten all the muscles of the body. Exhale. Repeat this sequence **2 more times**.

Authors' Recommendation: Deep relaxation. Sit at the back of the chair, relax completely for **10 minutes**.

Comments: This kriya gently works on the pituitary recharging your energy and reducing frustration and depression.

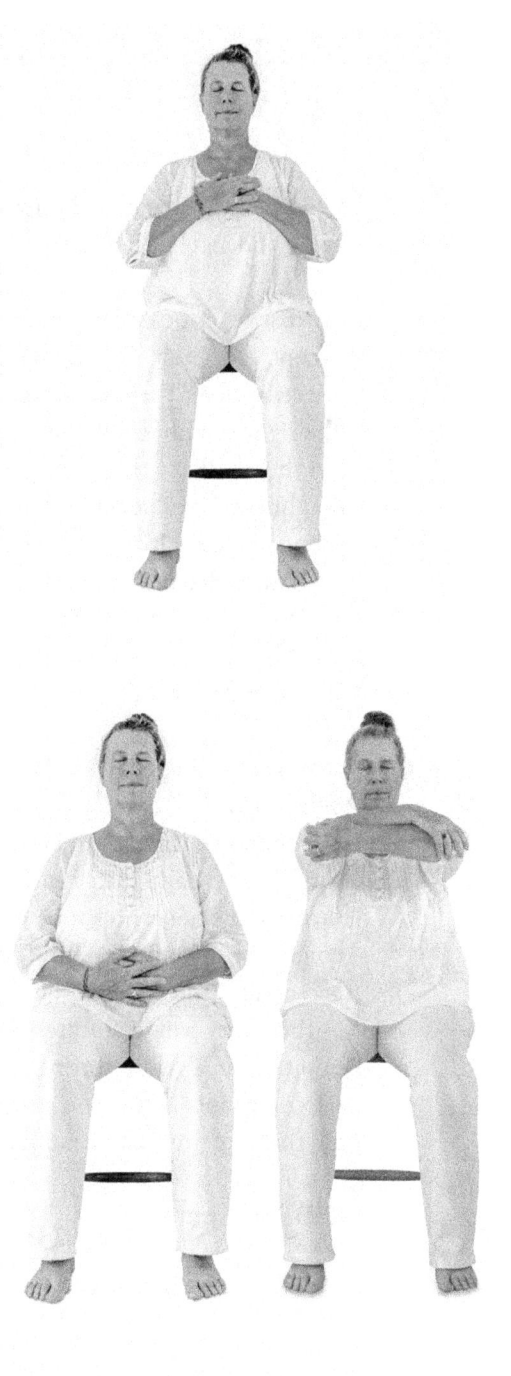

9.3 Meditation for Powerful Energy
May 17, 1976

Sit in Easy Pose with a straight spine and a light Neck Lock.

Mudra: Interlock all of your fingers except your Sun (ring) fingers, which are straight and pressed together. The right thumb locks down the left thumb. Place the mudra at diaphragm level, several inches (about 8 cm) in front of the body, with the Sun (ring) fingers pointing out and up at a sixty-degree angle.

Eye Focus: Closed.

Breath: Inhale deeply and chant **ONG** on a long exhalation (approximately **15 seconds**). The mouth is held slightly open, and the sound comes through the nose; no sound or air comes through the mouth. The sound is created at the back of the throat as the upper palate vibrates. When practiced in a group setting, each person chants in their own breath rhythm, creating a continuous sound.

Time: 8 minutes.

Comments: This meditation supports the thyroid and balances your energy. "Ong" is the sound of the sixth chakra, the center of consciousness and by chanting it you experience the joy of life. It is best to do this meditation when you have time to sleep afterwards or when you have a hard day to face.

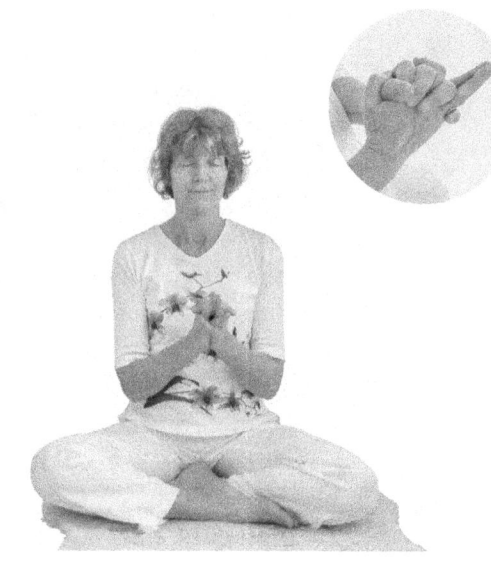

ON THE CHAIR

Sit comfortably in a chair with the weight of both feet resting evenly on the ground, with a straight spine, and a light Neck Lock.

Practice as described on the side.

Time: Start by chanting the mantra **3 times** and gradually build up to **4 minutes**.

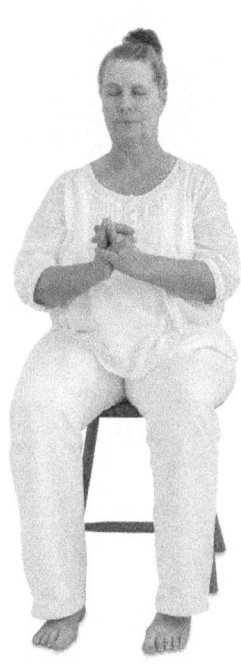

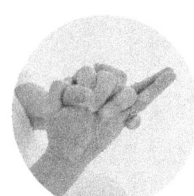

CHAPTER 10
Belonging

—

Live light, travel light, spread the light, be the light.
— YOGI BHAJAN, MAY 5, 1972

In this concluding chapter, you will work on the uppermost chakras, the seventh chakra, which represent the connection to the higher self, the realms of spirit and transcendence, and the energy of radiance. The seventh chakra is also known as the crown chakra or the Sahasrara. In this section you will work on your connection with where you came before your birth, your divine origin; experiencing bliss; being aware that you are being guided; being unattached; and not being afraid of death. In the uppermost chakra, the effects of all the chakras combine and are linked together.

The crown chakra is located above the skull. It has to do with your connection to what is higher, knowing that you are being guided, and thus protected. It also has to do with being detached, your spiritual growth, and experiencing bliss. Because you can befriend the unknown in the seventh chakra, you have the quality of being detached or unattached. The seventh chakra is where you experience unity and elevation, even to the level of enlightenment. This chakra is the command center of the nervous system, and the seat of the soul.

The seventh chakras' motto is: *I understand and I am free*. This chakra is associated with the color violet. There is no element. The organs are the cerebrum, the midbrain, and the pineal gland (also named the *epiphysis cerebri*).

Imbalances in this chakra can manifest as a sense of being cut off from a happy life, insecurity, sorrow, and also fear of death. With a weak seventh chakra, you can experience grief and disconnection from the abundance that life gives us.

What has an effect on your seventh chakra: Meditation; being in nature and absorbing it for a while; connecting with the infinite creative; being open to spiritual development; experiencing bliss.

As our life cycles on Earth come to an end, we prepare for the big letting go, the departure from this earth. The seventh chakra represents the connection with your higher source, the infinite creative. You can experience that we are we and we are one. It is critical to be grounded in order to experience this connection. It means that you must stand with both feet on the ground to avoid floating away. To be grounded connects us with our body, and with all the healing energy we have at our disposal in the present moment. As a result, you can feel the connection between earth and heaven's energy.

The kriya and meditation selected for this chapter focus on the connection between earth and heaven, grounding into the lower chakras and then elevating into the upper chakras and experiencing infinite awareness.

This section begins with pranayama or a breath practice called *Whistling Breath*. The whistling breath relaxes your system through the whistling vibration of the breath, which stimulates the vagus nerve. The first kriya *Foundation for Infinity* provides a foundation for connecting with the infinite while also ensuring that you are well-connected with the earth. This set makes clear that to experience boundlessness, you have to be well grounded in the physical world. The exercises in this set open, stretch, and strengthen the pelvic area, which is literally the base of your body. The meditation at the end of the set also builds a solid foundation that enables you to experience your connection with the earth by projecting the mantra in your navel center. If you subsequently project the sounds through your crown chakra, you can experience the radiance of the *Sahasrara* or Crown Chakra. The *Meditation into Being* expands your awareness and your sense of self integrating the finite and infinite dimensions of your being.

10.1 Whistling Breath
Originally published in Praana, Pranee, Pranayam

1) WHISTLING WHILE BREATHING IN. Pucker your lips, concentrate on the Third Eye Point, and breathe in through the mouth making a high-pitched whistle. Breathe out through the nose. Listen and focus to the sound of the whistle on the inhalation and on the soft sounds of the breath through the nose of the exhalation. Continue for **3-5 minutes**.

2) WHISTLING WHILE BREATHING OUT. Reverse the procedure: Inhale through the nose and exhale through puckered lips making a high-pitched whistle. Focus on the Third Eye Point and listen to the sound of the whistle on the exhalation. Continue for **3-5 minutes**.

Comments: The vagus nerve is the longest cranial nerve. Its name is derived from the Latin word for 'wandering,' because it wanders from the brain stem through the organs in the neck, chest, and abdomen. Thus it is involved in heart rate, intestinal peristalsis, sweating, movements of the mouth related to speech and that keep the larynx open for breathing. Each distinct movement of the lips stimulates the vagus nerve. Whereas, medically speaking, the vagus nerve is already a key element, in yoga its importance has certainly a double weight.

The technique of whistling for meditation is very simple and widely known. Physiologically, whistling breath changes the circulation; the lung capacity is increased as well. The nerves in the tongue activate the higher glands, such as the thyroid and parathyroid. It also takes tensions and stress away, bringing relaxation, and creating balance. Subtly, whistling breath neutralizes the energy, opening your connection to the Infinite realms.

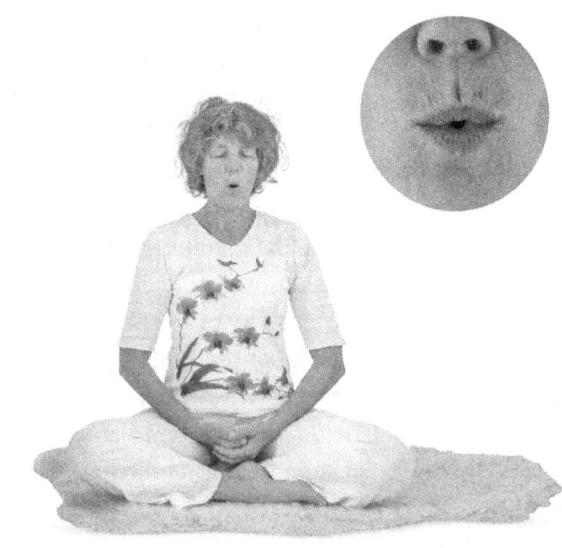

ON THE CHAIR

Sit comfortably in a chair with the weight of both feet resting evenly on the ground, with a straight spine, and a light Neck Lock.

Practice as described on the side.

Time: Start with **2 minutes** for each part and gradually build up to **5 minutes** each.

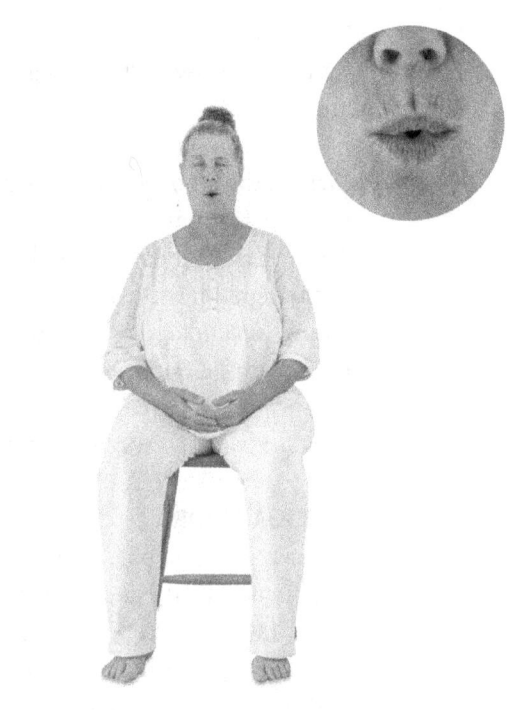

10.2 Kriya Foundation for Infinity
Originally published in The Aquarian Teacher Yoga Manual

1) SPINAL TWIST VARIATION.
Sit in Easy Pose with a straight spine and a light Neck Lock. Interlock the fingers behind the head at the hairline. Stretch the elbows out to the sides with the forearms parallel to the ground. Twist to the left on the inhale and twist to the right on the exhale. Keep the elbows up and open. (Do not reverse the breath.) Continue for **3 minutes**. *This helps remove tension from the shoulders and relaxes the chest muscles.*

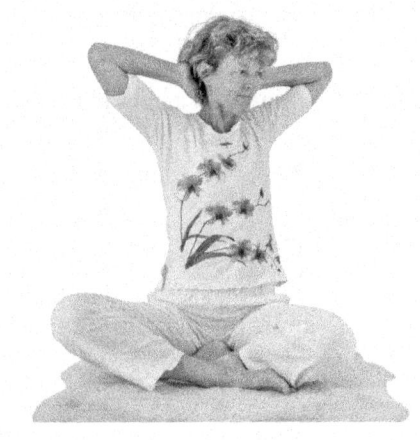

2) YOGA MUDRA.
Remain in Easy Pose. Interlace the fingers at the base of the spine, palms facing up. Bend from the hips, touching the Third Eye to the ground, and simultaneously raise the arms up behind the back. Rise back up. Create a steady rhythm alternating between these two positions in coordination with the breath. Continue for **2 minutes** with Breath of Fire.

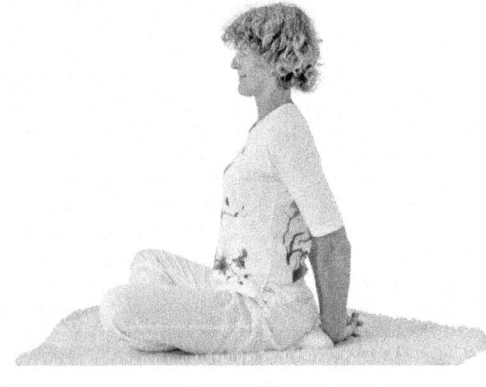

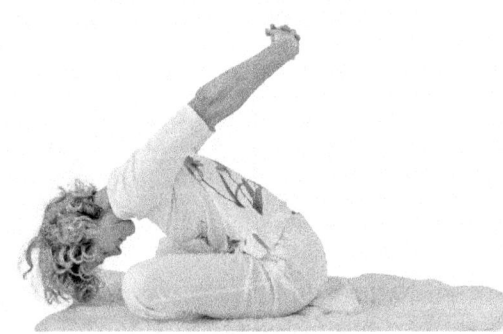

→ continue on next page

ON THE CHAIR

1) SPINAL TWIST VARIATION.
Sit comfortably in a chair with the weight of both feet resting evenly on the ground, with a straight spine, and a light Neck Lock. Interlock the fingers behind the head at the hairline. Stretch the elbows out to the sides with the forearms parallel to the ground. Twist to the left on the inhale and twist to the right on the exhale. Keep the elbows up and open. (Do not reverse the breath.) Start at a slow pace and increase it if possible. Continue for **1 ½ minutes**. *This helps remove tension from the shoulders and relaxes the chest muscles.*

2) YOGA MUDRA.
Remain seated with the feet hip-width apart with a straight spine. Interlace the fingers at the base of the spine, palms facing up. Bend from the hips and simultaneously raise the arms up behind the back. Rise back up. Create a steady rhythm alternating between these two positions in coordination with the breath. Continue for **1 minute** with Breath of Fire.

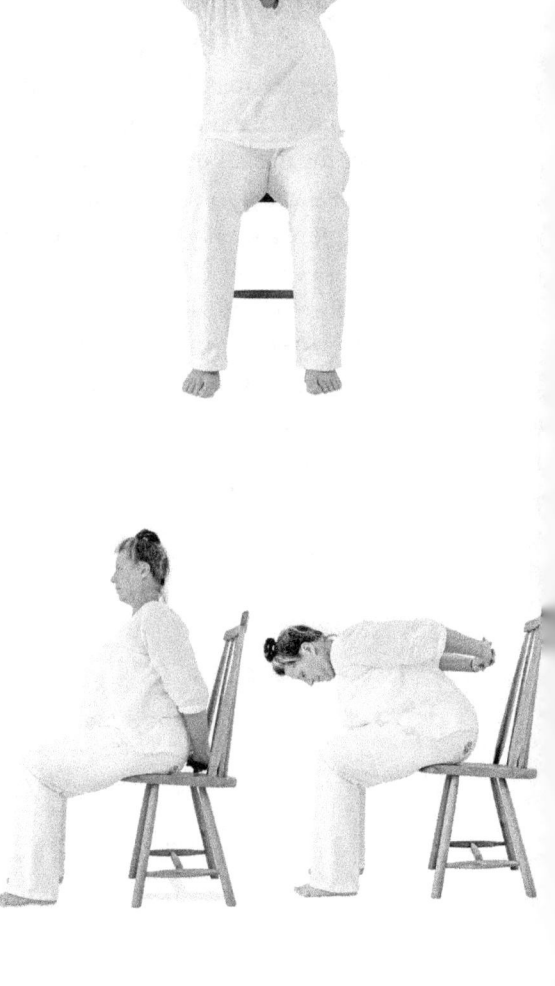

→ continue on next page

3) BACK PLATFORM POSE.

Sit with the legs stretched forward, feet together and toes pointed. Place the hands on the ground behind your hips, ideally fingers pointing forward. Apply Neck Lock, engage the Navel Point and lift the pelvis up until the body is in one long line from the toes to the crown of the head. Keep the Heart Center lifted and the Neck Lock applied to avoid compressing the back of the neck. Lower the buttocks to the ground to the starting position. Create a steady rhythm alternating between these two positions in coordination with the breath. Continue for **1 ½ minutes** with Breath of Fire. *This exercise increases the strength and flexibility of the pelvic area and releases the pelvis if it is locked.*

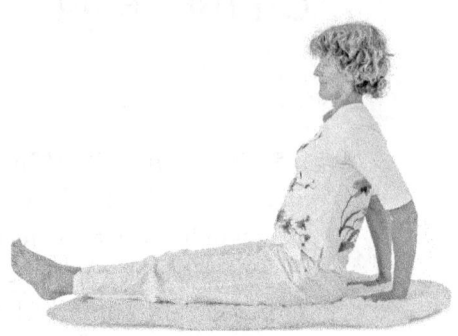

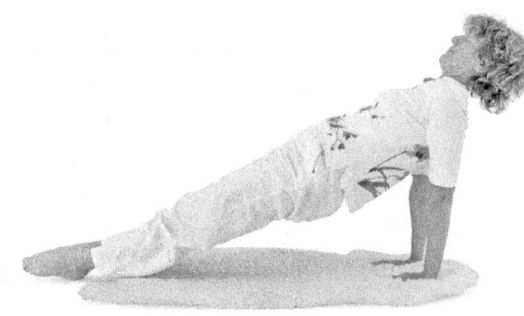

→ continue on next page

3) BACK PLATFORM POSE.

Remain seated slightly to the front of the chair. Stretch the left leg forward and the right foot flat on the ground. Apply Neck Lock, engage the Navel Point, grasp the sides of the chair and, if possible, lift the pelvis up. Keep the Heart Center lifted and the Neck Lock applied to avoid compressing the back of the neck. Lower the buttocks down on the chair to the starting position. Create a steady rhythm alternating between these two positions in coordination with the breath. If you cannot perform this movement, you can also visualize this. Continue for **45 seconds** with Breath of Fire. Then switch legs with the right leg stretched forward for **45 seconds**. *This exercise increases the strength and flexibility of the pelvic area and releases the pelvis if it is locked.*

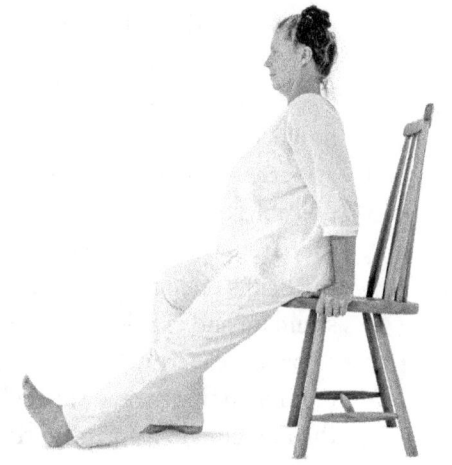

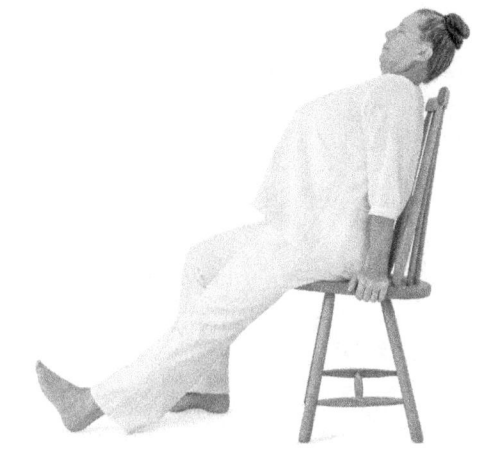

→ continue on next page

4) CROW SQUATS.

Stand up with the feet hip-width apart; knees, ankles, and feet are close to parallel alignment. Squat down, keep the spine elongated, and as perpendicular to the ground as possible. Stretch the arms straight forward parallel to the ground with the palms facing down. Inhale as you stand up and exhale as you squat down into a Crow Pose; hands stay parallel to the ground throughout the movement. Repeat **26 times**.

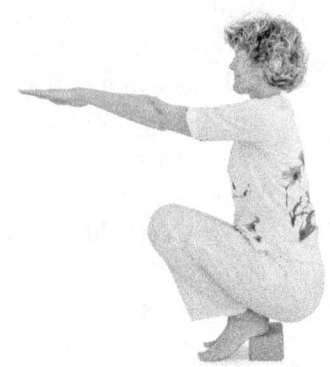

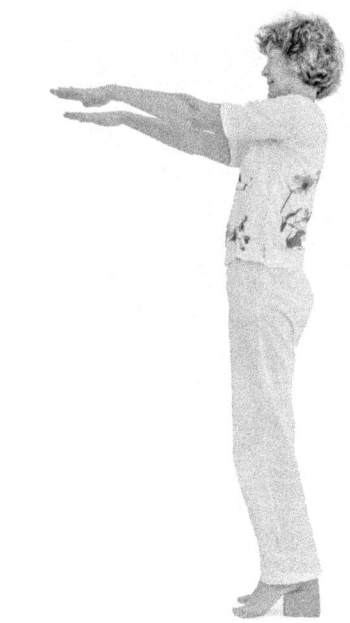

→ continue on next page

4) CROW SQUATS[1].

Remain seated with the feet hip-width apart and the spine straight. Stretch the arms forward. Inhale, raise the left knee up as if pulling your foot out of the mud. Exhale, and lower the foot down. Raise and lower alternate legs **13 times**.

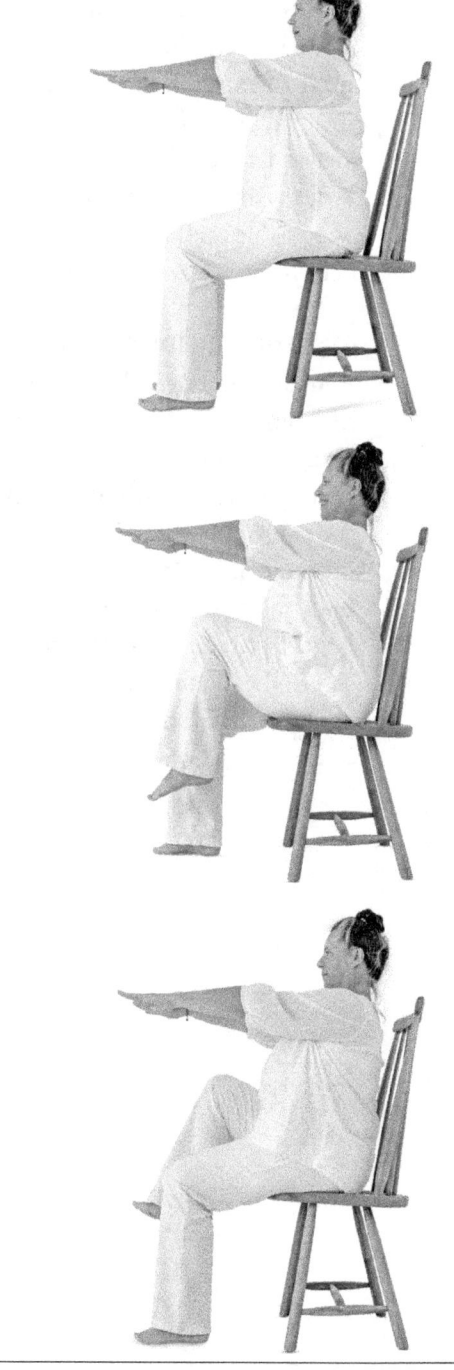

---

1 If standing, you can grab a chair or the edge of a table to maintain balance. Stand with the feet flat on the ground and equally distribute the weight to both feet. Lower your body as far as your knees allow. If the heels come up during the exercise, place a block or a rolled-up blanket under the heels. Make sure you stand on the entire sole of the foot, to be able to lower yourself with a straight back.

→ continue on next page

5) MIRACLE BEND VARIATION.
Stand up with the feet hip-width apart and stretch the arms up straight, palms facing forward. Bend forward, touch the ground on the exhale. Rise up and bend back as far as possible on the inhale, applying a light Root Lock. Repeat **26 times.**

6) STANDING SIDE STRETCH.
Remain standing. Inhale, elongate the spine, extend the right arm straight up and bend to the left, letting the left hand slide down the side of the body. Exhale, come up and bend to the right. Keep the body facing forward and alternate bending to each side **26 times**.
TO END: Inhale to the center, exhale, and relax.

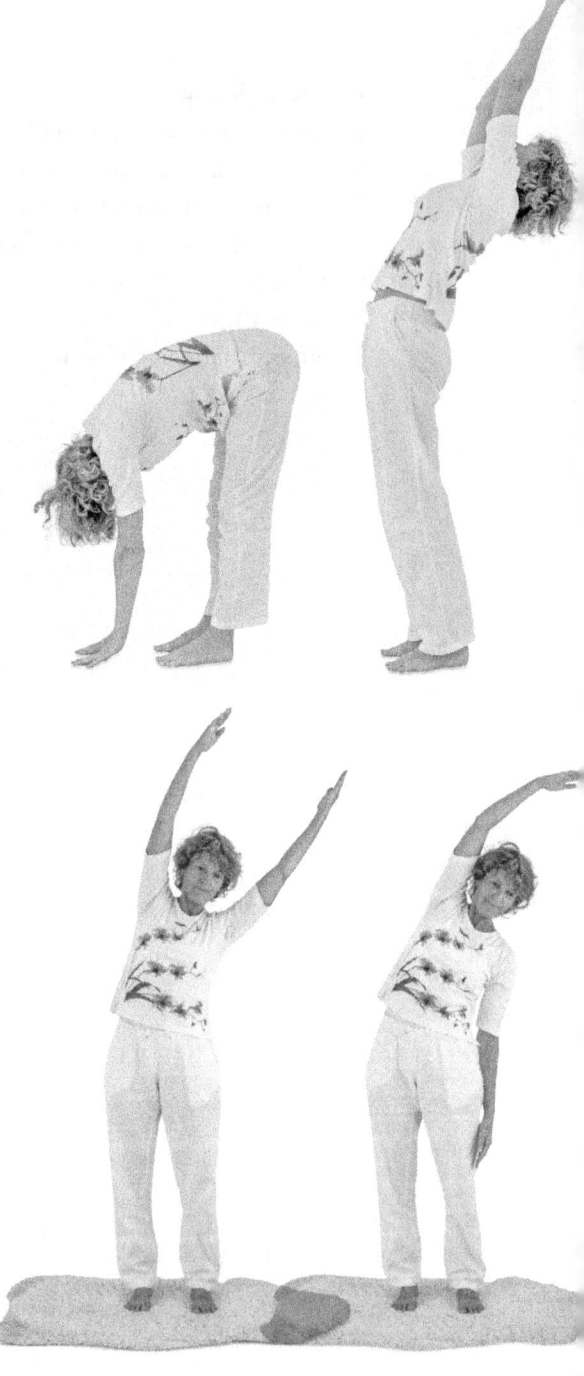

→ continue on next page

5) MIRACLE BEND VARIATION.
Remain seated with the feet hip-width apart and a straight spine. Activate the pelvic floor muscles and Navel Point, press the feet into the ground. Inhale, elongate the back and stretch both arms straight up, palms forward and slowly bend backward, keep the neck in line with the spine. Exhale, bend forward and then down. Create a steady rhythm moving between leaning backward and bending forward and down in coordination with the breath. Continue this cycle **13 times**.

6) SIDE STRETCH.
Remain seated. Inhale, elongate the spine, extend the right arm straight up and bend to the left, letting the left hand slide down the side of the body. Exhale, come up and bend to the right. Keep the body facing forward and bend **13 times to each side**.
TO END: Inhale to the center, exhale, and relax.

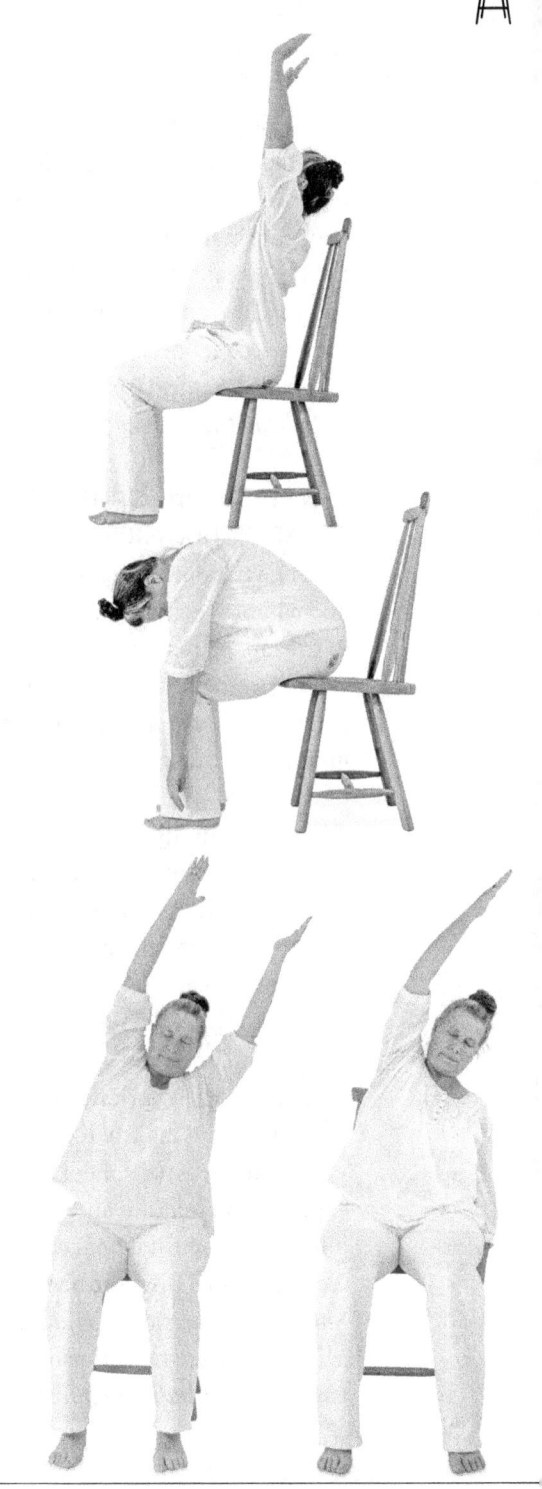

→ continue on next page

7) YOGIC KICKS.

Remain standing with the feet closer together. Place the hands on the hips. Kick alternate legs forward, keeping the legs straight. Chant **HAR** with each kick. Continue rhythmically 1 kick per second for **3 minutes**.
A common tendency is to kick too quickly or to bend the knee when kicking.

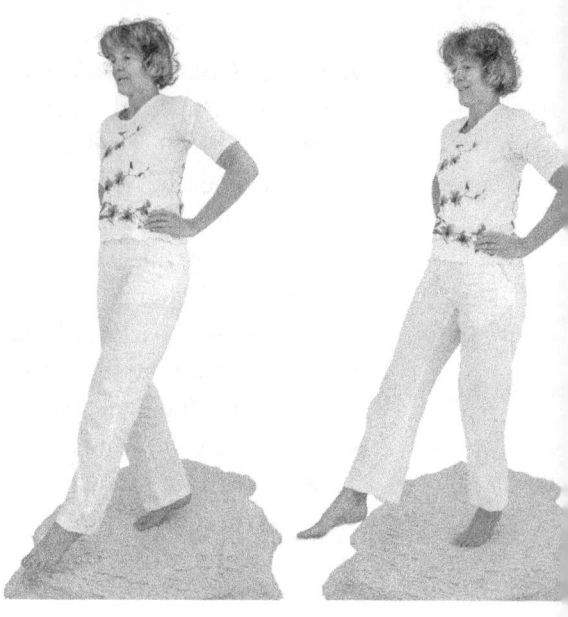

8) MEDITATION FOR THE TENTH GATE: TO EXPERIENCE YOUR BOUNDLESSNESS.

Sit in Easy Pose with a straight spine and a light Neck Lock. Place the hands in the lap, palms facing up, right palm resting in the left, pads of the thumbs touching. Focus the eyes upward, guiding the attention to the top center of the head—the Tenth Gate or Crown Chakra. Mentally vibrate the mantra **HAR HAR** as you pull the Navel Point in. Holding the navel in, press the tip of the tongue against the roof of the mouth and mentally say the word **MUKANDAY**. Concentrate deeply and immerse yourself in this meditation to experience the radiance of the Crown Chakra. Experience your boundlessness. Feel yourself expand beyond time and space, into a realm of total peace and joy. Continue for **11-31 minutes**.
Singh Kaur's version of Har Har Mukanday from the Crimson Series works well with this meditation.

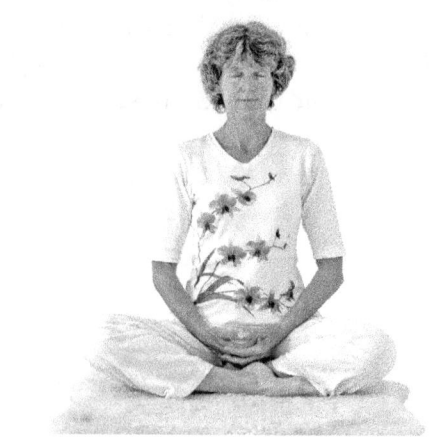

→ continue on next page

7) YOGIC KICKS.
Remain seated, slightly forward on the chair. Place the feet part way forward and place the hands on the waist and kick alternating legs forward, while keeping the legs straight. Chant **HAR** with each kick. Continue rhythmically 1 kick per second for **1 ½ minutes**.

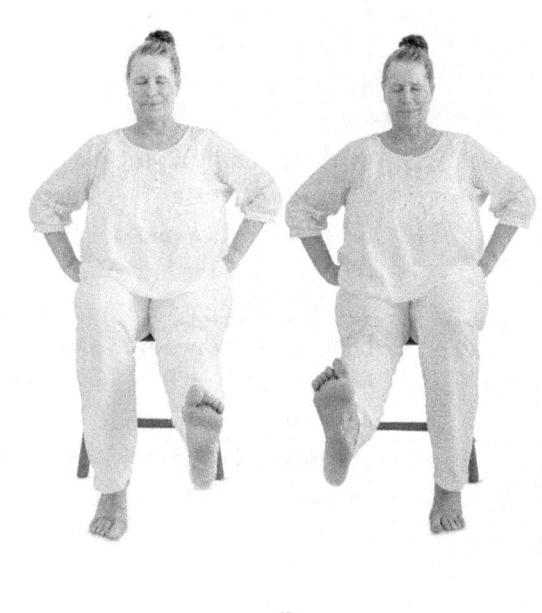

8) MEDITATION FOR THE TENTH GATE: TO EXPERIENCE YOUR BOUNDLESSNESS.
Remain seated with the feet hip-width apart, with a straight spine, and a light Neck Lock. Place the hands in the lap, palms facing up, right palm resting in the left, pads of the thumbs touching. Focus the eyes upward, guiding the attention to the top center of the head—the Tenth Gate or Crown Chakra. Mentally vibrate the mantra **HAR HAR** as you pull the Navel Point in. Holding the navel in, press the tip of the tongue against the roof of the mouth and mentally say the word **MUKANDAY**[2]. Concentrate deeply and immerse yourself in this meditation to experience the radiance of the Crown Chakra. Experience your boundlessness. Feel yourself expand beyond time and space, into a realm of total peace and joy. Continue for **3-11 minutes**.

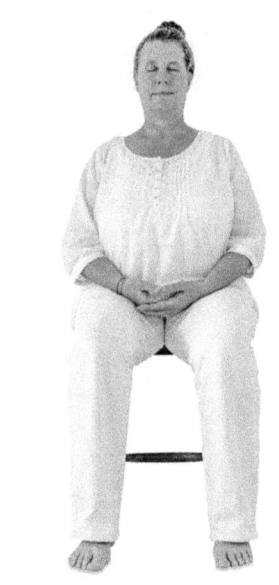

---

2 Authors' Note: The mantra Har Har Mukanday supports liberation and letting go of sorrows. Har empowers and develops willpower, and Mukanday means liberator.

→ continue on next page

Comments: To reach the subtle realm of ether where we are by nature boundless, we must first set a firm foundation on Earth. This kriya works primarily on the pelvic region. Physiologically the pelvis acts as a foundation, the point of balance for the torso and the lower extremities. The female pelvis is especially delicate, because the bones aren't fused together, and are therefore easily misaligned. Chronic misalignment, tension, and inflexibility will eventually show their effects physically and emotionally in both men and women.

Singh Kaur's version of Har Har Mukanday from the Crimson Series works well with this meditation.

Comments: To reach the subtle realm of ether where we are by nature boundless, we must first set a firm foundation on Earth. This kriya works primarily on the pelvic region. Physiologically the pelvis acts as a foundation, the point of balance for the torso and the lower extremities. The female pelvis is especially delicate, because the bones aren't fused together, and are therefore easily misaligned. Chronic misalignment, tension, and inflexibility will eventually show their effects physically and emotionally in both men and women.

10.3 Meditation into Being: I Am I Am
April 7, 1972

Sit in Easy Pose with a straight spine and a light Neck Lock.

Mudra: Relax the right hand in Gyan Mudra on the right knee, keeping the elbow straight. Raise the left hand 6 inches (15 cm) in front of the Heart Center with the palm facing the chest and the fingers pointing to the right. Chant **I AM** and emphasize **"I"** as you draw the hand closer to 4 inches (10 cm) in front of the Heart Center. Chant **I AM** and emphasize **"AM"** as you move the hand straight out from the body to 12 inches (30 cm) at the Heart Center level. Take a breath and return the hand to the original position of 6 inches (15 cm) in front of the Heart Center.

Eye Focus: 1/10th open, look straight ahead through the eyelids.

Breath: Inhale as you draw the hand into the original position 6 inches (15 cm) in front of the Heart Center, exhale naturally as you chant. Create a steady rhythm with the mantra and the breath.

Mantra: I AM, I AM.

Time: 11-31 minutes.

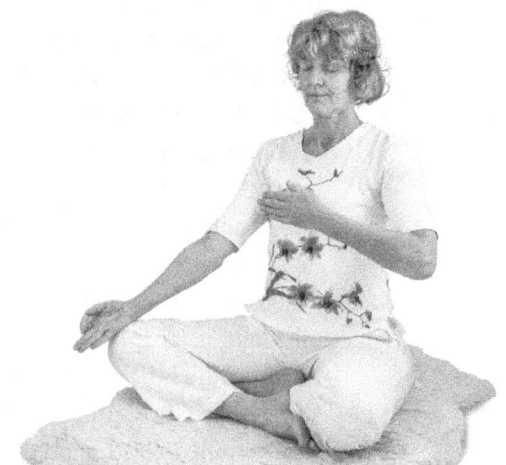

→ continue on next page

ON THE CHAIR

Sit comfortably in a chair with the weight of both feet resting evenly on the ground, with a straight spine, and a light Neck Lock.

Practice as described on the side.

Time: Start with **3 minutes** and gradually build up to **11 minutes**.

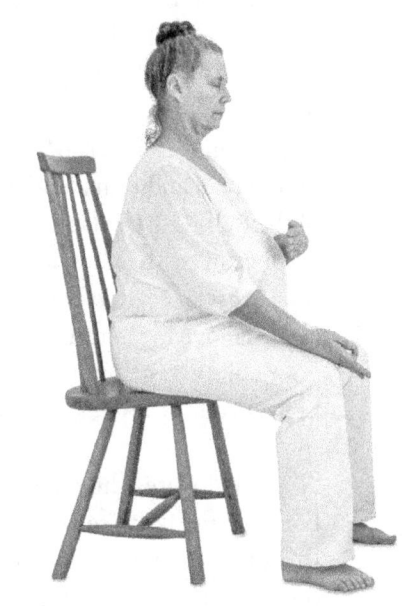

To End: Inhale deeply, suspend the breath, exhale, and relax.

Comments: This mantra connects the finite and infinite identities, and dissolves duality. The first "I Am" emphasizes the "I," the personal and finite sense of self. The second "I Am" slightly emphasizes the "Am," the impersonal and transcendent sense of the Self. To be what you are is the essence of truth and will lead you to the nature of reality. The hand and the breath move in rhythm and strengthen your ability to maintain a sense of Self as your awareness expands.

A yogi cultivates the relationship between the finite sense of the self and the infinite sense of the Self. The mind often forgets this relationship when it becomes attached to a particular emotion or object that it wants to keep. One of the important habits the yogi instills in the mind is the ability to break that trance of attachment by shifting the perspective from the individual to the Infinite. This is also the perspective of Being. You exist before the objects you collect and even before the body that you use. It is very powerful and effective to remind the mind of your true identity with your Infinite Being. What the yogi seeks is to participate in life with authenticity and wholeness.

CHAPTER 11
Additional Resources – Self-Care Kit

So you have done all this work to better take care of yourself, as well as your boundaries, your needs, and internal listening. You have worked on the seven chakras focusing on your foundations, enjoyment, self-esteem, awareness, self-expression, sense of purpose, and belonging. You reached this far and have consistently come back for your own self. This is the work to keep you rooted in the present moment, connected to your body, and with all healing energy you have at your disposal at the present moment.

In this extra chapter, you may connect with your aura and your radiance. The aura is one of your ten bodies and is also, in the Kundalini Yoga as taught by Yogi Bhajan, your eighth chakra. The eight chakra concerns what you project and what protects you. It is also responsible for the health of the immune system. Nothing more appropriate for a Self-Care kit, ending a program that it's all about taking better care of yourself. The eighth chakra, along with the seventh, connect us with infinity and with our higher self, and the seed of our self, the soul. Through these two chakras you can realize your own completeness and connection with all that is.

The eight chakras' motto is: *I radiate and I am protected*. The eighth chakra has the ability to absorb energy, information, and either allow it to pass or block it. A strong aura gives us confidence and support no matter where we are. The electromagnetic field, which is measurable, serves as the foundation of the aura. It surrounds the body in the same way that the earth is surrounded. You need strong nerves and a strong magnetic field to be happy. This chakra is associated with the color white. There is no element. There are no organs. The aura ensures that all chakra effects are linked.

11.1 Warm-Up with Butterfly

You can choose one or more of these as a warm-up before practicing the kriyas presented in this book.

1) POINT AND FLEX FEET.
Sit with a straight spine and both legs straight forward. Place the hands on the lap or on the thighs. Alternately, stretch the feet forward and pull the feet backward (a full cycle lasts 1-2 seconds). Continue for **1 minute**.
This exercise stimulates circulation through the legs and feet, and strengthens the muscles in the lower legs.

2) YOGI MARCH.
Stand straight, weight evenly distributed on both feet with the arms by your sides. Connect with the earth and find your balance. Bend the elbows with the hands at shoulder height in Gyan Mudra, palms facing forward. Inhale, lift your left knee as high as possible, and simultaneously stretch both arms straight up; exhale, lower the foot and arms. Repeat with the other knee. Create a rhythmic movement for **1 minute**.

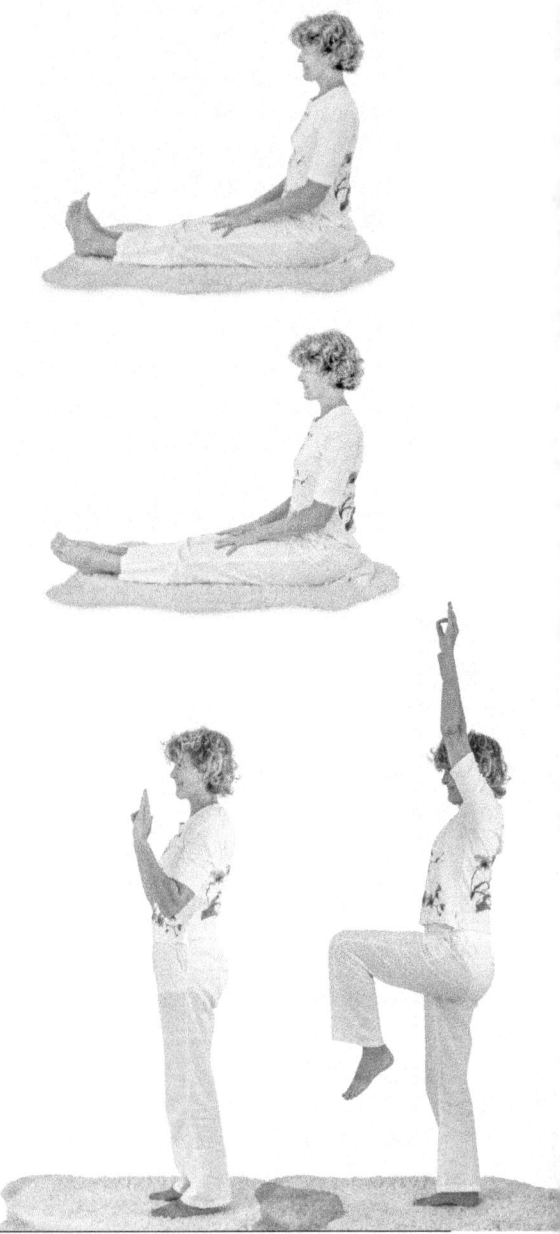

→ continue on next page

ON THE CHAIR

1) POINT AND FLEX FEET.
Sit comfortably in a chair, feet hip-width apart and even weight on both feet with a straight spine and a light Neck Lock and the hands on the thighs. Lift the heels and return the feet flat on the ground. Continue for **30 seconds**. Then keep the heels on the ground and lift the feet and return back down for **30 seconds**.

2) YOGI MARCH.
Remain seated with a straight spine. Inhale, lift the left knee and simultaneously stretch both arms straight up, hands in Gyan Mudra; exhale, lower the knee and arms. Repeat with the other knee. Create a rhythmic movement alternating legs for **1 minute**.

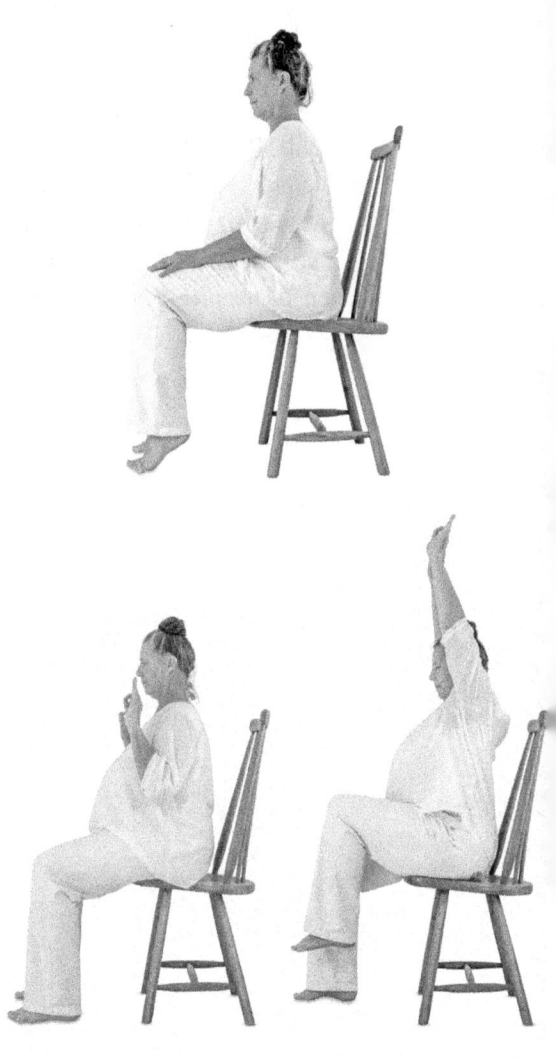

→ continue on next page

3) BUTTERFLY.

Sit with a straight spine and a light Neck Lock. Bring the soles of the feet together, knees out to the sides. Wrap the hands around the feet or grasp the ankles drawing the heels as close to the groin as possible. Keep the spine elongated with a light Neck Lock. Move your knees up and down for **1 minute**. *This posture opens the hips and is beneficial for sitting in Easy Pose.*

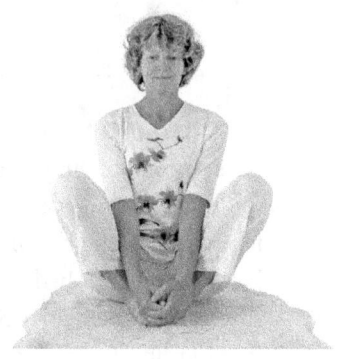

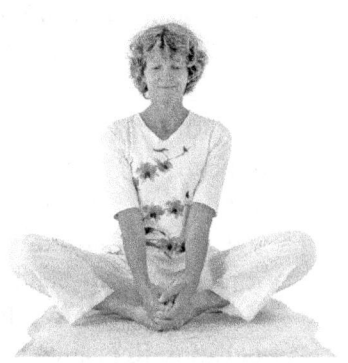

3) BUTTERFLY.

Sit slightly to the front of the chair. Bring the soles of the feet together, if possible. Grab the edge of the chair. Elongate the back and apply a light Neck Lock. Move the knees up and down for **6 times**.

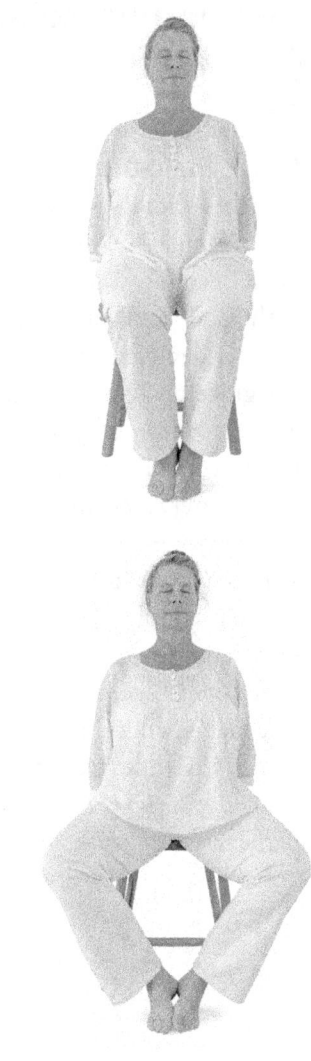

11.2 Movement Relaxation Series
August 22, 1986

1) RHYTHMIC DANCE.
Stand up with a straight spine and arms completely relaxed. Close the eyes. Become aware of any tension in the body and consciously let it go. Sway and move every part of the body in a graceful dance. Gentle, rhythmic elevating music may be played. Dance with ease for **3-11 minutes.** Immediately start the next exercise.

2) BODY AWARENESS.
Remain standing with closed eyes. Use your hands to lightly feel every part of the body. Every square inch must be touched with the sensitivity of the palms. Continue for **3-5 minutes.**
Touching the body confirms the reality of the relaxation and smooths the aura.

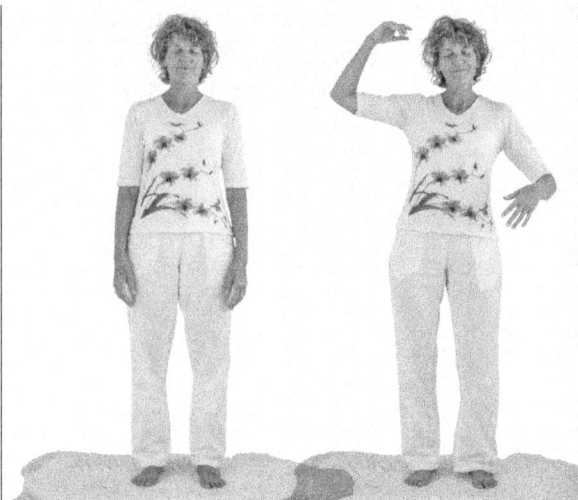

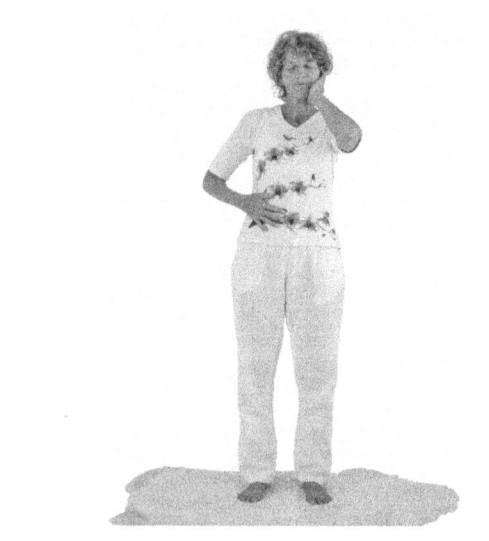

→ continue on next page

ON THE CHAIR

1) RHYTHMIC DANCE.
Sit comfortably in a chair with the weight of both feet resting evenly on the ground, with a straight spine and a light Neck Lock. Close the eyes. Become aware of any tension in the body and consciously let it go. Sway and move every part of the body in a graceful dance. Gentle, rhythmic elevating music may be played. Dance with ease for **1-3 minutes.** Immediately start the next exercise.

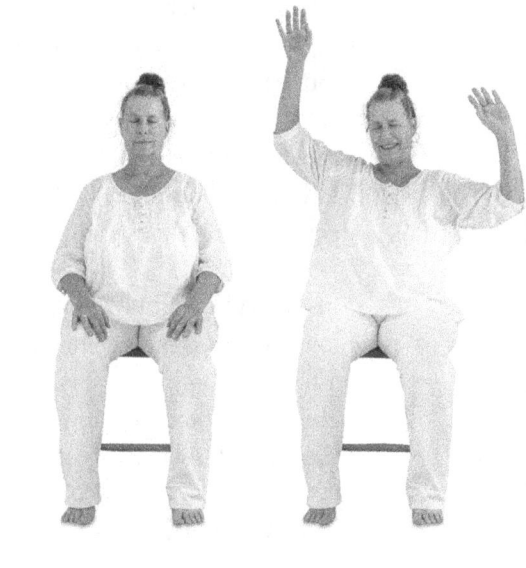

2) BODY AWARENESS.
Remain seated with a straight spine and closed eyes. Use your hands to lightly feel every part of the body. Every square inch must be touched with the sensitivity of the palms. Continue for **1-3 minutes.** *Touching the body confirms the reality of the relaxation and smooths the aura.*

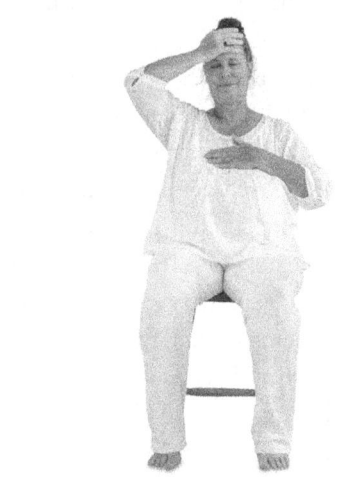

→ continue on next page

3) HANGING RELAXATION.

Remain standing, lean forward from the hips, go down only as far as the arms can hang loosely (the fingers or hands may not reach the ground). Completely relax the head, neck and arms. Continue for **3-11 minutes** with normal breathing. TO END: Inhale and exhale deeply several times.

4) BACKWARD RELAXATION.

Slowly rise up and lean backwards with arms hanging loosely behind the body. Continue for **1 minute** with relaxed breath.

5) RELAXATION.

Lie on the back in Corpse Pose and completely relax for **10 minutes**.

Comments: The rhythmic free movement in this meditative kriya relaxes and releases the physical and mental tension caused by stress, which is built up over time. Some of the exercises strengthen the heart and circulatory system. When this system is weak, the tissues become tense and the joints build up deposits that may lead to illness, and make it difficult for the body to deeply relax. When the body can totally relax and the mind and body act cooperatively, you can experience the Self.

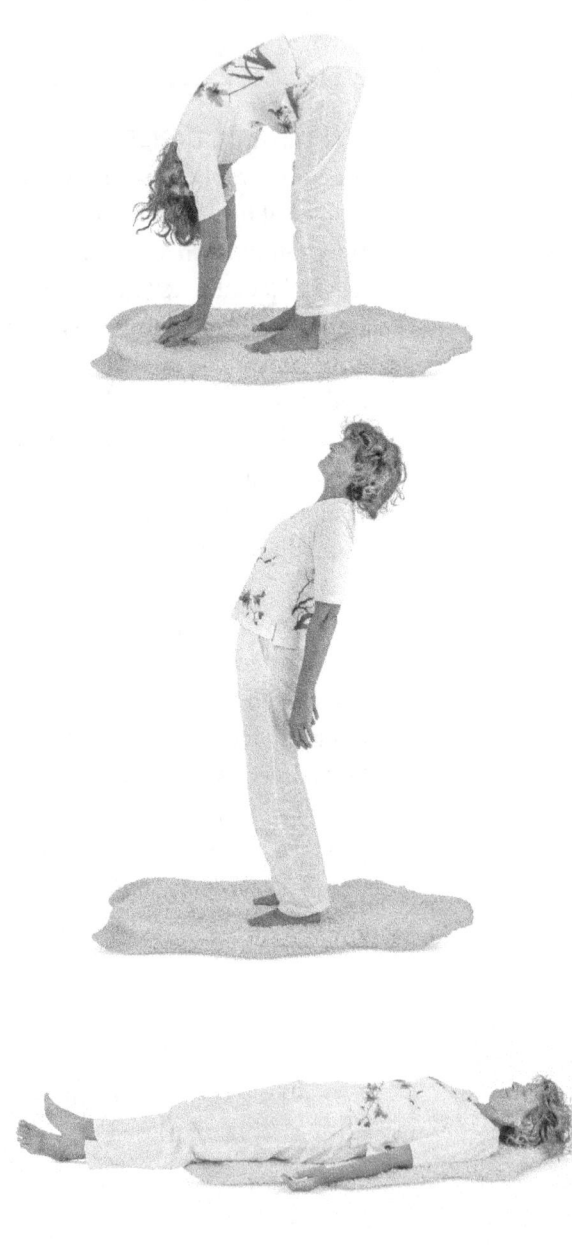

3) FORWARD BEND.

Remain seated with a straight spine. Lean forward from the hips, go down only as far as the arms can hang loosely (the fingers or hands may not reach the ground). Completely relax the head, neck and arms. Continue for **1-3 minutes** with normal breathing. TO END: Inhale and exhale deeply several times.

4) BACKWARD BEND.

Remain seated. Elongate the back and slowly bend backward, keep the neck in line with the spine and relax the arms down behind the back. Continue for **1 minute.**

5) RELAXATION.

Sit with the feet comfortably apart on the ground and connect with the earth. Relax the hands on the upper legs, palms up. Continue for **3-10 minutes**.

Comments: The rhythmic free movement in this meditative kriya relaxes and releases the physical and mental tension caused by stress, which is built up over time. Some of the exercises strengthen the heart and circulatory system. When this system is weak, the tissues become tense and the joints build up deposits that may lead to illness, and make it difficult for the body to deeply relax. When the body can totally relax and the mind and body act cooperatively, you can experience the Self.

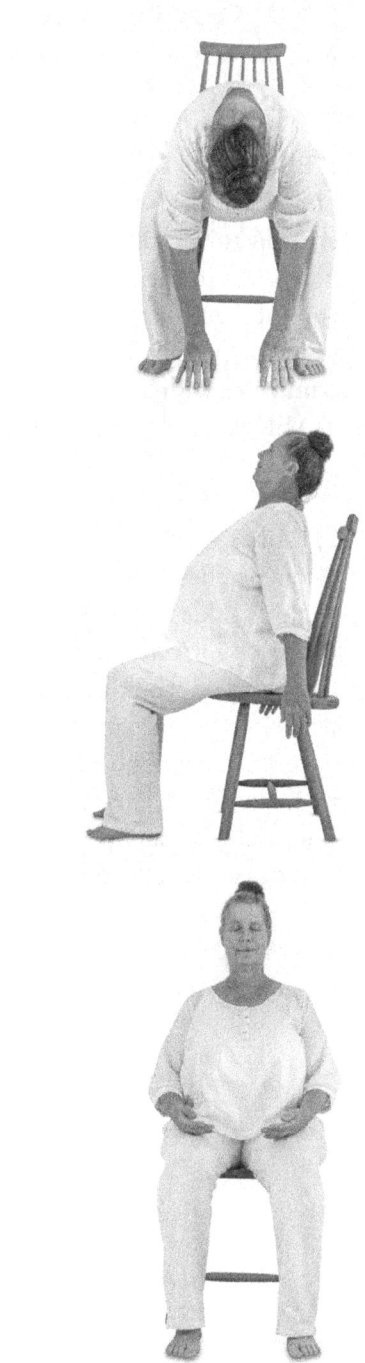

11.3 Kriya for the Electromagnetic Field

Originally published in Aquarian Times, Summer 2003

1) BREATH OF FIRE.
Sit in Easy Pose with a straight spine and a light Neck Lock. Place the hands on the knees in Gyan Mudra (tips of thumbs and index fingers touch.) Maintain this posture for **3 minutes** with Breath of Fire.
TO END: Inhale, suspend the breath for a few seconds, exhale, and relax.

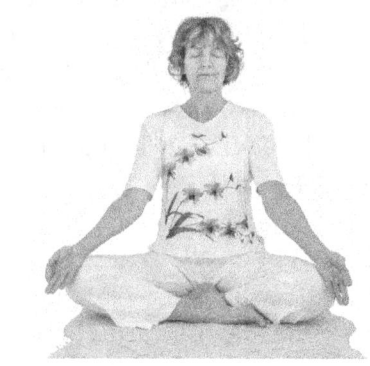

2) CAMEL RIDE.
Remain in Easy Pose. Grasp the shins or ankles with the hands. Tilt the pelvis forward on the inhale and backward on the exhale. Only the pelvis and lower spine move. The rib cage, shoulders, and head are still and remain over the hips. The motion is fluid and continuous. Continue for **3 minutes**. Breathe powerfully.
TO END: Inhale, elongate the spine, suspend the breath for a few seconds, exhale, and relax.

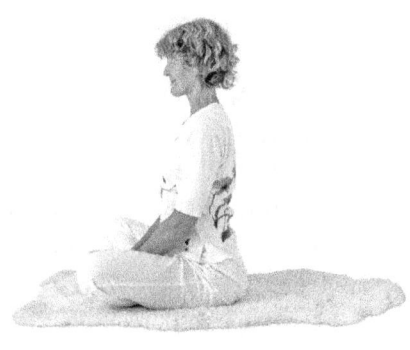

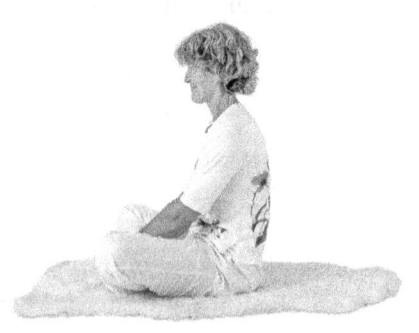

→ continue on next page

ON THE CHAIR

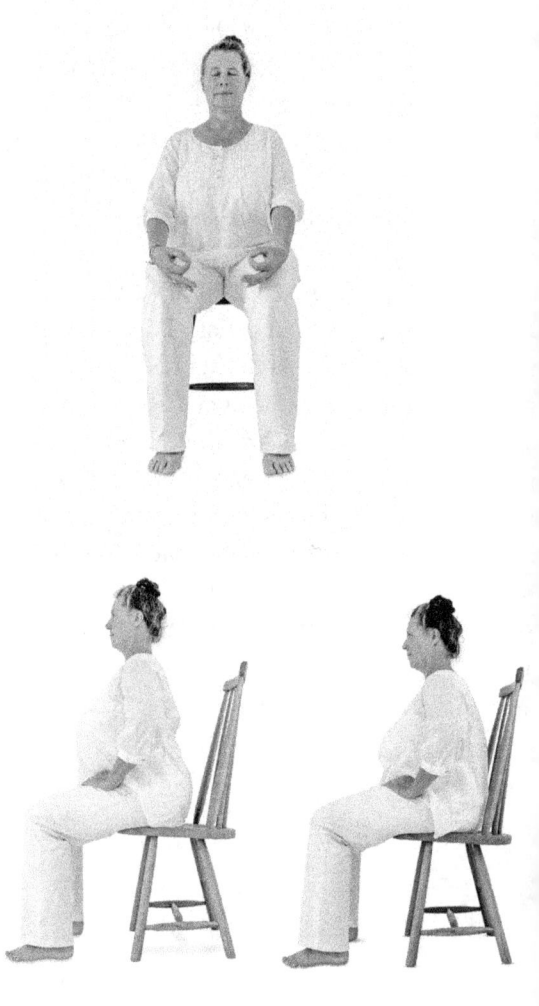

1) BREATH OF FIRE.
Sit comfortably in a chair, feet hip-width apart and even weight on both feet with a straight spine and a light Neck Lock. Place the hands on the knees in Gyan Mudra (tips of thumbs and index fingers touch.) Maintain this posture for **1 minute** with Breath of Fire.
TO END: Inhale, suspend the breath for a few seconds, exhale, and relax.

2) CAMEL RIDE.
Remain seated with the feet hip-width apart and a straight spine. Place the hands on the upper thighs at the crease of the hips. Tilt the pelvis forward on the inhale, and backward on the exhale. Only the pelvis and lower spine move. The rib cage, shoulders, and head are still and remain over the hips. The motion is fluid and continuous. Continue for **1 minute**. Breathe powerfully.
TO END: Inhale, elongate the spine, suspend the breath for a few seconds, exhale, and relax.

→ continue on next page

3) NAVEL PRESS.

Remain in Easy Pose and press the tip of the right thumb into the navel. Continue for **3 minutes** with Long Deep Breathing.
TO END: Inhale deeply, exhale completely, suspend the breath, and press the thumb firmly into the navel for a few seconds. Then inhale and relax.

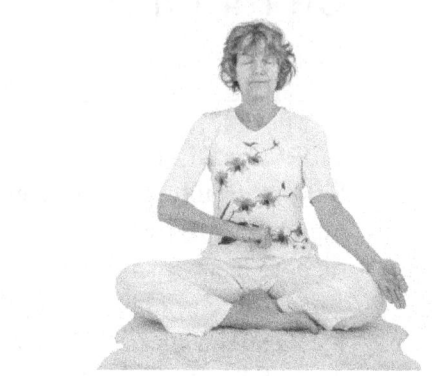

4) SHOULDER SHRUGS.

Remain in Easy Pose with a straight spine and a light Neck Lock, and grasp the knees. Raise both shoulders up towards the ears on the inhale, drop the shoulders down on the exhale. Continue for **3 minutes**. Move and breathe powerfully.
TO END: Inhale and raise the shoulders, hold for a moment, exhale, lower the shoulders, and relax.
The exercise relaxes the shoulders, neck, and upper back.

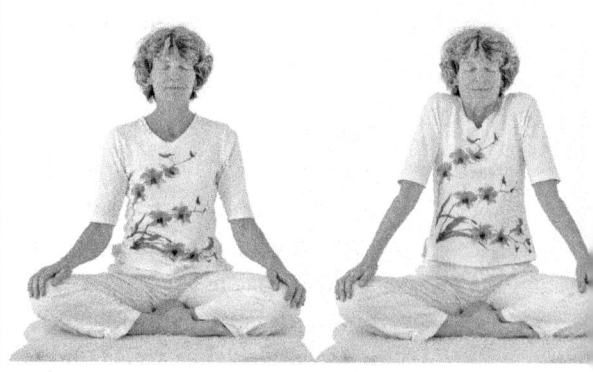

→ continue on next page

3) NAVEL PRESS.

Remain seated with the feet hip-width apart and a straight spine. Press the tip of your right thumb into the navel. Continue for **1 minute** with Long Deep Breathing.
TO END: Inhale deeply, exhale completely, suspend the breath, and press the thumb firmly into the navel for a few seconds.
Then inhale and relax.

4) SHOULDER SHRUGS.

Remain seated with the feet hip-width apart and a straight spine. Place the hands on the thighs, keep the arms straight. Raise both shoulders up towards the ears on the inhale, lower the shoulders on the exhale. If you have a shoulder injury, move with care. Continue for **1 minute**.
TO END: Inhale and raise the shoulders, hold for a moment, exhale, lower the shoulders, and relax.
The exercise relaxes the shoulders, neck, and upper back.

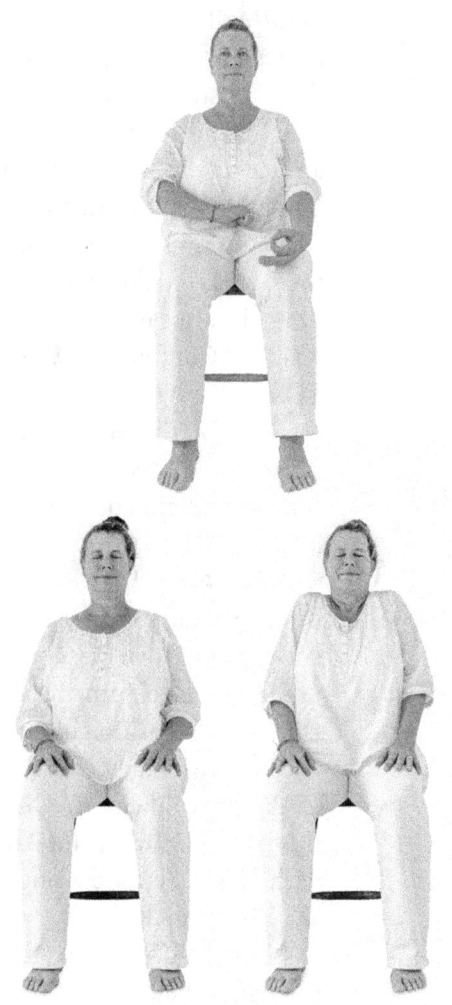

→ continue on next page

5) ARM CIRCLES.

Remain in Easy Pose and stretch the arms straight forward with the palms facing each other. Inhale and swing the arms back as far as possible, palms facing forward. Keep the arms stretched and swing them back and down. Exhale and bring the arms back to the starting position. Continue for **3 minutes**.
TO END: Inhale deeply with the arms held in the back position, suspend the breath for a few seconds, exhale, and relax.

6) MEDITATE.

Remain in Easy Pose with eyes slightly open focusing at the Tip of the Nose. Relax the hands in a comfortable position on the knees or in the lap. Mentally chant **WHAA-HAY** on the inhale and **GUROO** on the exhale. Continue for **3 minutes** with Long Deep Breathing.
TO END: Inhale deeply, suspend the breath for a few seconds, exhale, and relax.

Comments: The electromagnetic field surrounds your body in the same way the Earth's magnetic field envelops the Earth. The electromagnetic field is also called the aura, and, when it is strong, it attracts positive energy and protects us from negativity and illness.

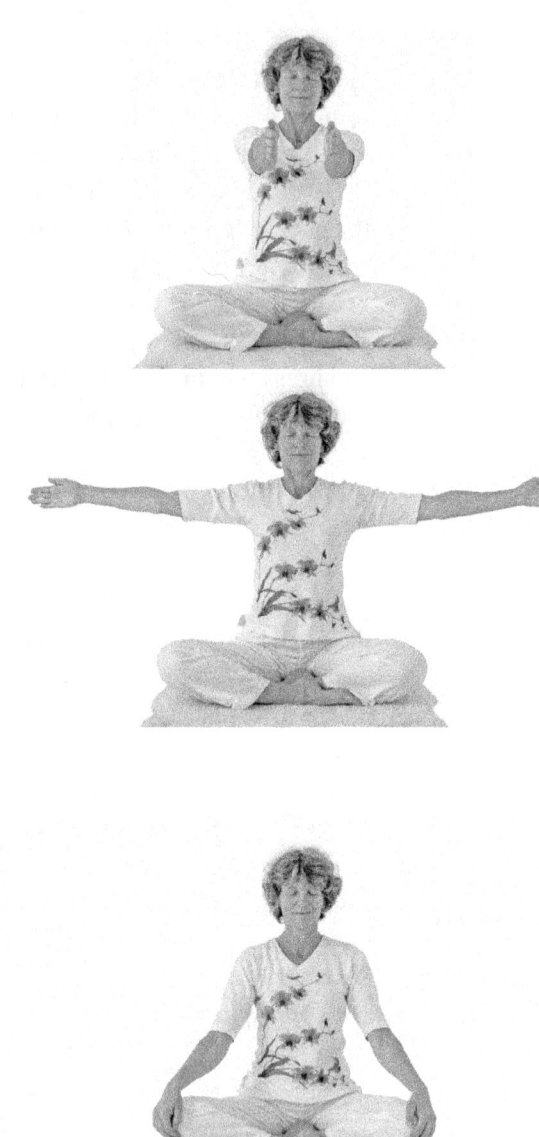

5) ARM CIRCLES.
Remain seated with the feet hip-width apart and a straight spine. Stretch the arms straight forward with the palms facing each other. Inhale and swing the arms back as far as possible, palms facing forward. Keep the arms stretched and swing them back and down. Exhale and bring the arms back to the starting position. Continue for **1 minute**.
TO END: Inhale deeply with the arms held in the back position, suspend the breath briefly. Exhale and relax.

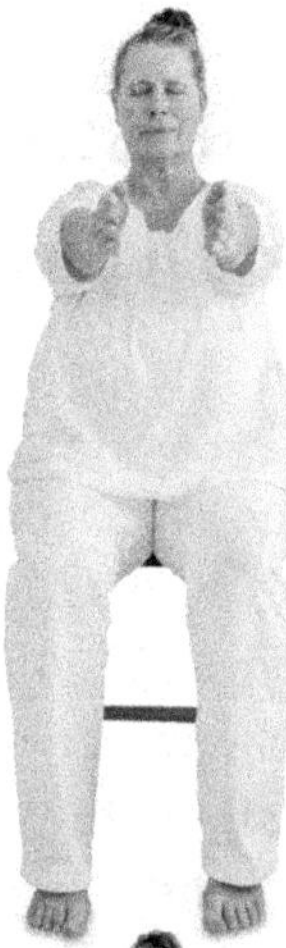

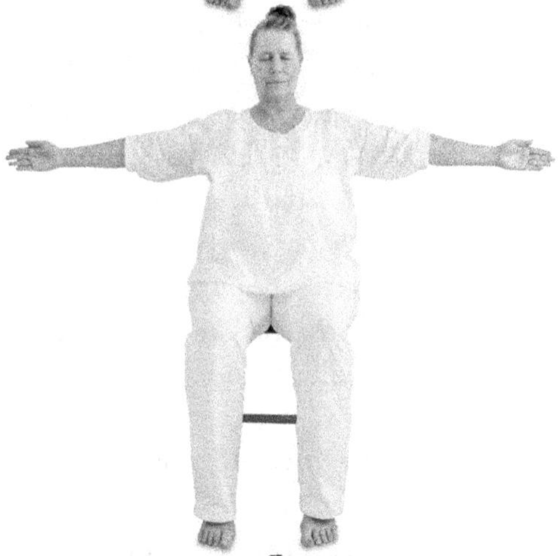

6) MEDITATE.
Remain seated with the feet hip-width apart and a straight spine with eyes slightly open focusing at the Tip of the Nose. Relax the hands in a comfortable position on the knees or in the lap. Mentally chant **WHAA-HAY** on the inhale and **GUROO** on the exhale. Continue for **1 minute** with Long Deep Breathing.
TO END: Inhale deeply, suspend the breath briefly, exhale, and relax.

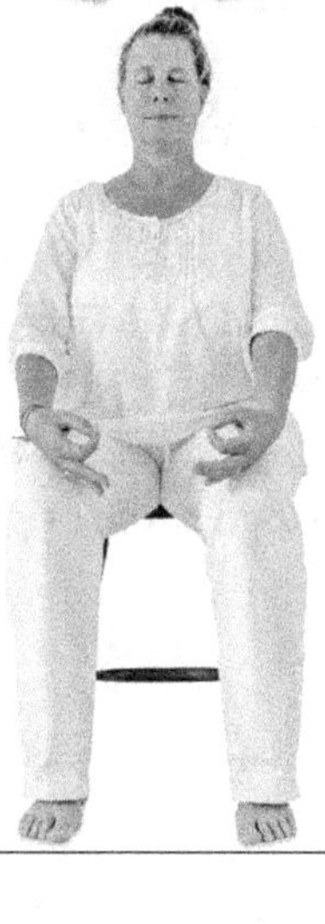

Comments: The electromagnetic field surrounds your body in the same way the Earth's magnetic field envelops the Earth. The electromagnetic field is also called the aura, and, when it is strong, it attracts positive energy and protects us from negativity and illness.

11.4 Meditation for the Arcline and to Clear the Karmas
August 1, 1996

Sit in Easy Pose with a straight spine and a light Neck Lock.

Mudra: Rest the elbows at the sides of the body. Extend the forearms forward parallel to the ground with hands facing up slightly cupped. Keeping the elbows bent, raise the arms up and back over the shoulders as far back as possible on each "WHAA-HAY GUROO" and "WHAA-HAY JEEO." Immediately return to the starting position (1 cycle per 2 seconds). The movement is as if scooping water and throwing it with a flick of the wrists over the shoulders and through the arcline.

Eye Focus: Closed.

Breath: Not specified.

Mantra: Listen to the mantra: **WHAA-HAY GUROO, WHAA-HAY GUROO, WHAA-HAY GUROO, WHAA-HAY JEEO.** ("Wahe Guru, Wahe Guru, Wahe Guru, Wahe Jio" by Gyani Ji was played in the original class.)

Time: 31 minutes.

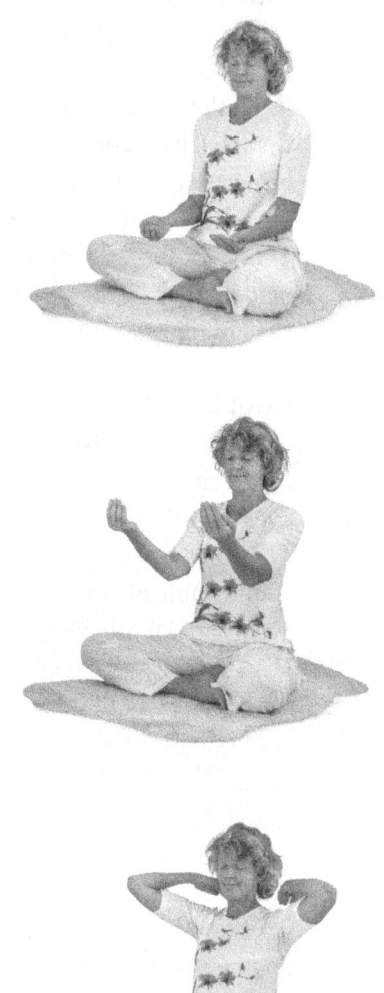

→ continue on next page

ON THE CHAIR

Sit comfortably in a chair with the weight of both feet resting evenly on the ground, with a straight spine and a light Neck Lock.

Practice as described on the side.

Time: Practice for **3-5 minutes**.

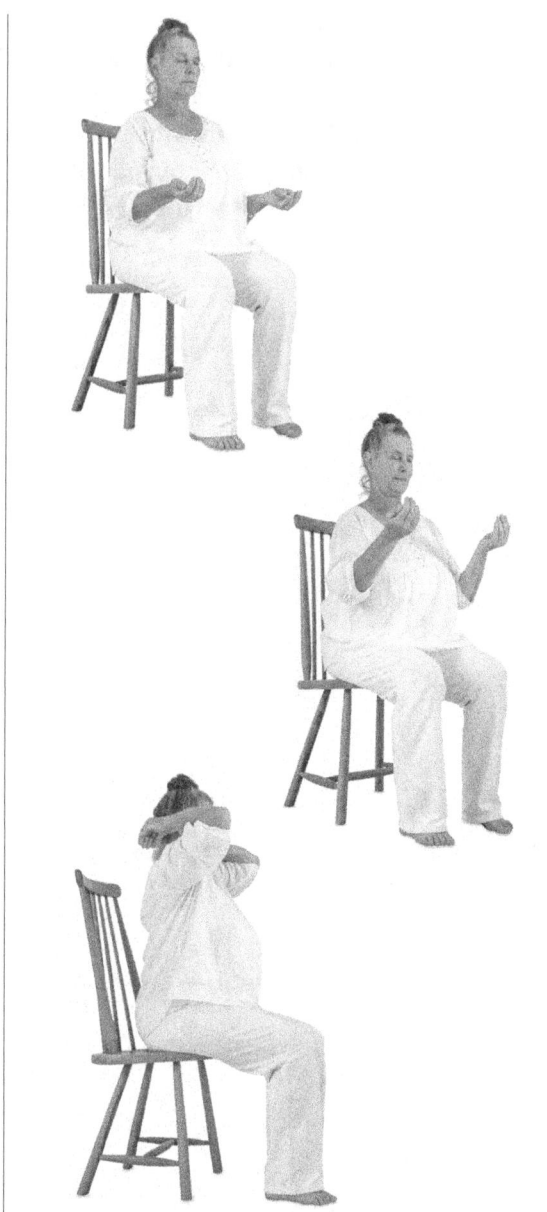

To End: Inhale deeply, stretch the hands as far back as possible, suspend the breath **10-15 seconds**, exhale. Repeat **2 more times**.

Comments: This meditation is said to clear karmic memory that is held within the arcline. The power of Infinity is within you, not outside of you.

11.5 Become Calm – Earth to Self
January 31, 1996

Sit in Easy Pose with a straight spine and a light Neck Lock.

Mudra: Make fists with both hands with the Jupiter (index) fingers extended and the other fingers held down with the thumbs. Synchronize the movements with the mantra. With the arms straight, touch the ground by the sides of the body on "Sat" and "Whaa-Hay." Bend the arms and touch the tips of the Jupiter fingers in front of the chin on "Naam" and "Guroo." One complete cycle takes **6-7 seconds**. Concentrate, so that the fingertips touch.

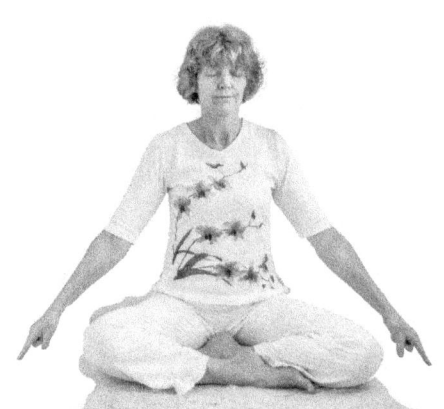

Eye Focus: Closed.

Breath: Not specified.

Mantra: SAT NAAM SAT NAAM, WHAA-HAY GUROO WHAA-HAY GUROO. (In the original class, "Sat Nam Wahe Guru #2," by Jagjit Singh was played.)

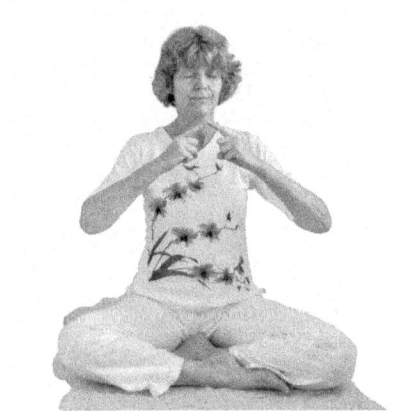

Time: 3 minutes.

Comments: When you are very tense, do this and you will become calm, quiet, peaceful, and tranquil.

ON THE CHAIR

Sit comfortably in a chair with the weight of both feet resting evenly on the ground, with a straight spine and a light Neck Lock.

Practice as described on the side.

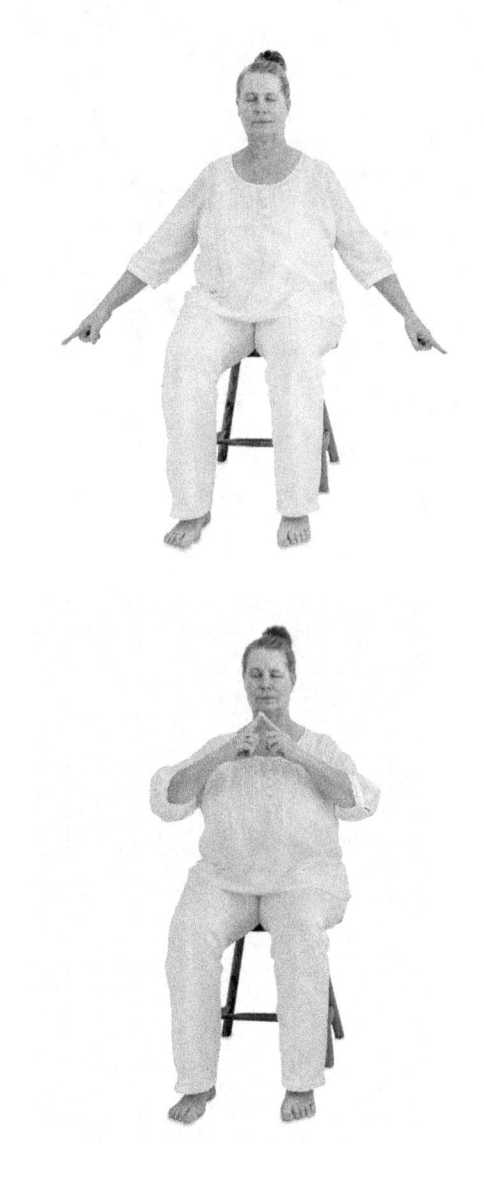

ABOUT THE AUTHORS

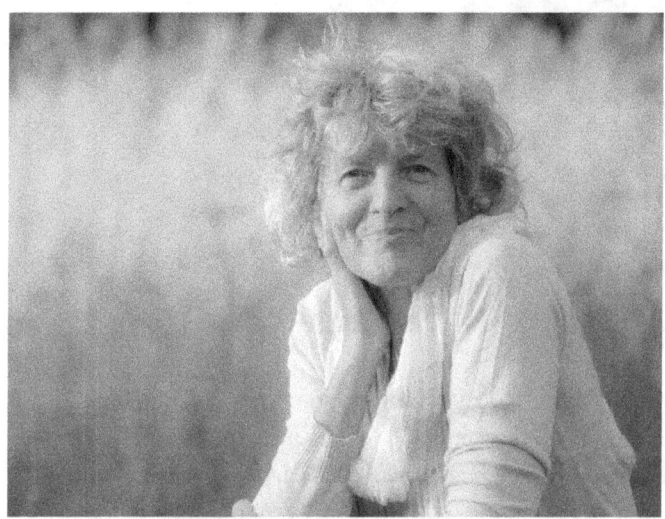

photo credit: Rita Punt

Ivonne Wopereis has been a yoga practitioner for 19 years. In 2007, she began her Kundalini Yoga Teacher Training in Thailand and finished it in 2010 at Yogacentrum Michon in Enschede, Netherlands. In 2011, she advanced her training by completing the Level Two module "Stress and Vitality," which helped her better identify and handle stress issues using Kundalini Yoga practices.

Aside from stress and vitality, the elderly and vulnerable people have always been her primary interests. She attended the *Fachausbildung Yoga für Senioren* in Germany in 2014, where she studied specific strategies for teaching yoga to the elderly and vulnerable communities. To enhance her education, she attended Guru Ram Das Center seminars with Atma Jot and Dr Shanti Shanti Kaur Khalsa on several modules of Yoga as Therapy. She began her studies in Sat Nam Rasayan in Amsterdam in 2016 in order to operate more intuitively, and she has attended various courses both at home and abroad. She has been teaching Kundalini Yoga since 2007 and designing chair adaptations of Kundalini Yoga programs since 2011.

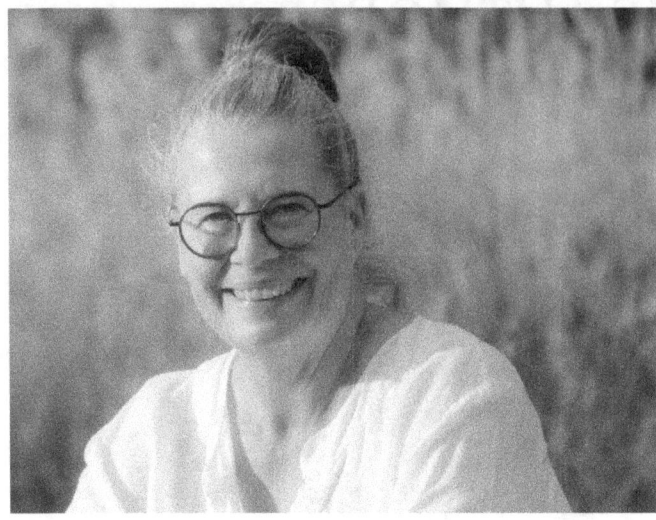

photo credit: Rita Punt

Monique Siahaya, also known as Amrit Kriya Kaur, graduated from Kundalini Yoga Teacher Training in 1988 and has been teaching yoga ever since. She completed the Sivananda pregnancy yoga training in The Hague in 1990 as part of her development, and she finished her Kundalini Yoga training with the Level Two modules in the following decades. To focus even more on therapeutic yoga, she has learned Sat Nam Rasayan and completed several segments of Yoga and Therapy with Atma Jot and Dr Shanti Shanti Kaur Khalsa from the Guru Ram Das Center for Medicine & Humanology. She has recently begun to learn how to play the gong for relaxation.

She met people who couldn't sit on the floor or stand for lengthy periods of time due to aging or disease while conducting regular Kundalini yoga lessons. As a result, she began to develop yoga variations for the chair, so that people of advanced age or illness might benefit from Kundalini Yoga practice as well. She has been teaching yoga on a chair in nursing homes since 2002. Her passions and areas of competence include yoga for the elderly, chair yoga, and pregnancy. In 2011, she and fellow kundalini yoga teachers in Germany created the *3HO Fachausbildung für Senioren*, a professional training course specialized in yoga for the elderly.

She has experienced firsthand how practicing yoga and meditation can help one relax and be in control through stressful personal times or while caring for others. She has also worked with caregivers who say that yoga helps them and is important to them. For Monique, yoga is a way of life that connects you to the inexhaustible source of wisdom and light, allowing you to grow, understand better, accept more, and become happier. Yoga is the way to connect with your soul.

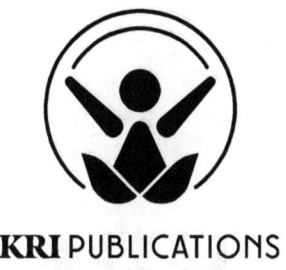

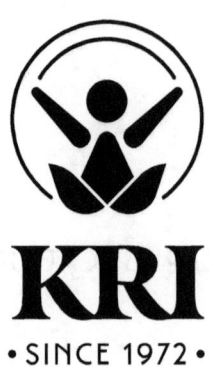

KUNDALINIRESEARCHINSTITUTE.ORG

www.ingramcontent.com/pod-product-compliance
Lightning Source LLC
Chambersburg PA
CBHW060531010526
44110CB00052B/2570